food for fit and
Healthy
kids

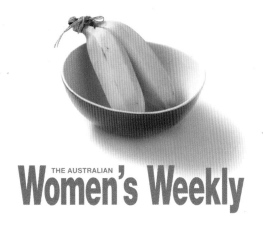

THE AUSTRALIAN
Women's Weekly

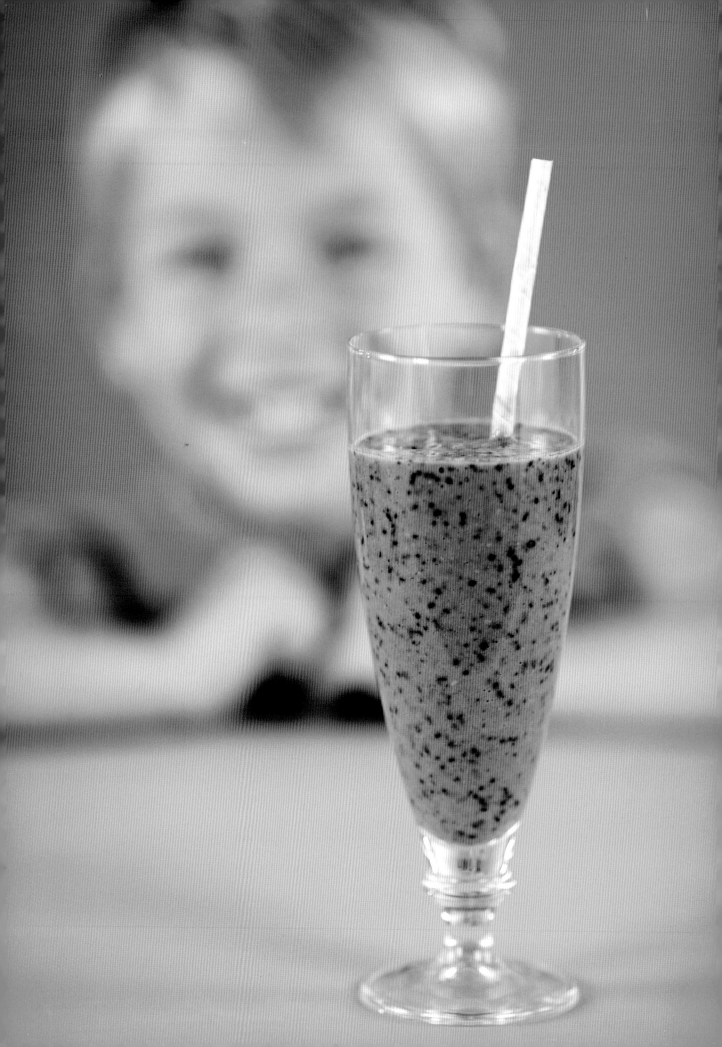

contents

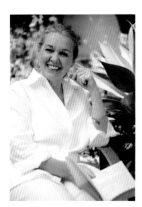

The childhood obesity debate is a complex and multi-faceted issue, but one aspect of it seems quite clear to me, and that's that good and healthy eating patterns have to begin at home. Parents must teach their children about nutrition through example: parents decide what's brought home from the supermarket, what goes in the lunchbox and what's served up at a hasty family breakfast. We hope this book helps guide you toward teaching your children healthy and appealing eating habits that they are eager to adopt for life.

Pamela Clark

Food Director

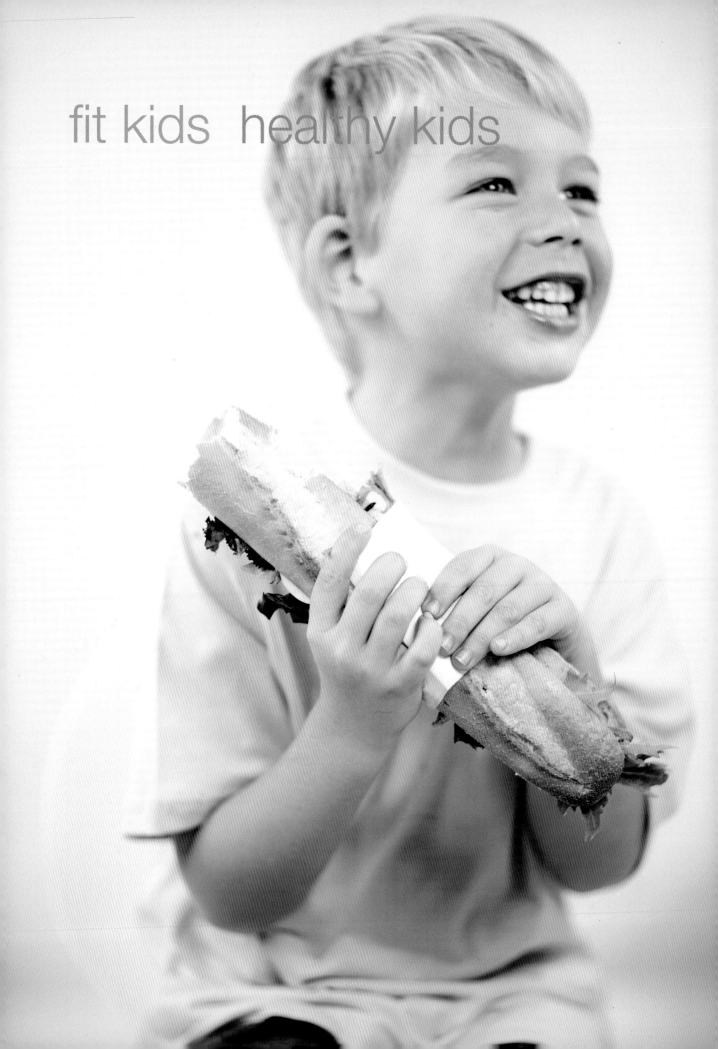

fit kids healthy kids

Welcome to *Food for Fit & Healthy Kids*. There's no better place to start than a cookbook when it comes to **advice** on how to get your kids into **healthy eating** and an active lifestyle.

Fundamentally, food starts in the home and revolves around family. From the rush at **breakfast** to a **snack** after school, the **kitchen** is the **hub of the home,** and the place where many of life's lessons are learned.

Most parents want the best for their children, and understand the basic principles of a **healthy lifestyle,** but turning this theory into **practical solutions** is the challenge, especially in today's fast-paced world. *Food for Fit & Healthy Kids* is a **practical** guide to getting things back on the health track. As role models it's about inspiring and nourishing the young ones in your life, but this book is about looking after **mums and dads too,** with great family recipes and smart strategies for a **healthy lifestyle for the whole family,** now and well into the future.

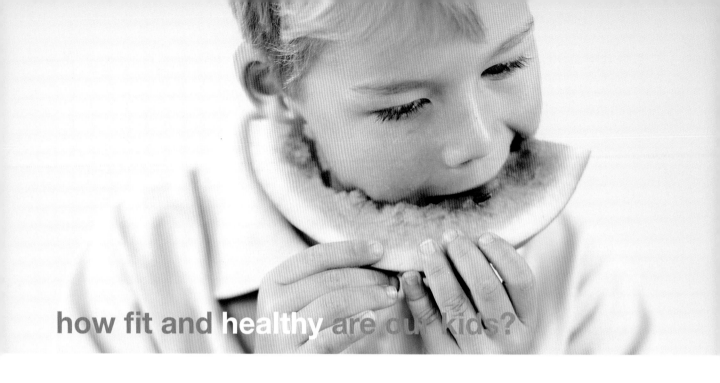

how fit and healthy are our kids?

battle of the bulge

With so much news concerning kids' health, especially the obesity debate, it's easy to imagine we are losing the battle of the bulge. The statistics around childhood obesity are alarming, however, it's important to realise that currently only one in four Australian and New Zealand children fall into the overweight or obese category. And, on average, kids are not fairing that badly in the fitness stakes. It's the rate of increase in the numbers becoming overweight that is the concern, with trends showing a faster pace in the last 20 years.

So, as a parent you are more than likely to have children who are currently of a healthy weight. The key is to keep them that way, faced with all of the challenges of what health professionals call the "obesogenic" environment. This basically refers to an environment that pushes us to eat more high fat, high sugar and kilojoule-laden foods; at the same time it's an environment that takes away the need to expend energy for daily activities. It's not hard to find food at anytime of the day or night in the obesogenic environment. Supermarkets are open extended hours, fast food restaurants are on every corner and you can dial for pizza from the comfort of home. Today we rely on timesavers such as computers, remote controls, dishwashers and automatic garage doors, and we use up far fewer kilojoules taking these easier options. Therefore, it's not hard to see how previous generations kept in shape – their diet was based on more healthy, whole foods and they simply had to move a lot more to get through their day.

self-assessment task

A great place to start to assess your child's healthy lifestyle is to look at how much physical activity they do per day. Keep a clock on their total screen time spent in front of the TV or computer. Getting the balance right with these two areas is fundamental to keeping a healthy weight.

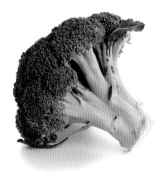

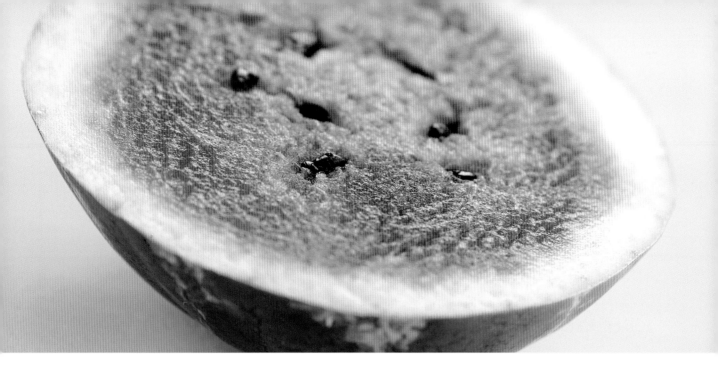

The official government Physical Activity Recommendations for Children and Youth state that:

1 Children and young people (from 5-18 years of age) should participate in at least 60 minutes of moderate to vigorous physical activity each day.

2 Children and young people should not spend more than two hours per day using electronic media for entertainment (e.g. computer games, internet, TV) particularly during daylight hours.

dietary deficiencies

Despite living with an abundant food supply, it's surprising to still see dietary deficiencies in some children. Even though children are generally getting enough food in total, they may be eating too many foods with poor nutrition quality, and not always reaching targets for particular food groups and essential nutrients like iron, calcium and zinc. This can affect their optimal growth and development today, but can also increase their risk of lifestyle diseases in the future. For example, calcium from dairy foods is vital for building strong bones and healthy teeth in children, and sufficient dietary calcium is needed every day to prevent bone thinning and osteoporosis in adult life. So it's no surprise one study has indicated that nearly one in four children who avoid milk will sustain a bone fracture.

Changing lifestyles can also bring about some unexpected changes to vitamin status in children. For example, there are new concerns about vitamin D status in kids. Vitamin D is vital for bone health and is mainly obtained from sunlight along with some food sources. It seems our best intentions of slip, slop, slapping our kids against harmful UV rays, may also be reducing their vitamin D status. There are now calls to fortify more foods with vitamin D to counteract this lifestyle change. Regular nutrition surveys and ongoing research is vital to help health professionals plan what is the optimum diet for kids in our changing world.

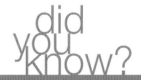

did you know?

Contrary to urban myths, watermelon seeds are oily and edible. According to the *Oxford Companion to Food*, the Chinese are particularly fond of eating the seed after removing the black shell.

self-assessment task

One of the easiest and fastest checks to assess the quality of your child's diet, is to write down everything they eat for a day and compare this with the recommended servings of the different food groups as stated in *The Australian Guide to Healthy Eating*. This will help you see if their diet is balanced and address any areas of shortfall. Sample serves from *The Australian Guide to Healthy Eating* suggested for children and adolescents are outlined below.

food groups	children 4-7 years	children 8-11 years	adolescents 12-18 years
bread, cereals, rice, pasta, noodles	3-4	4-6	4-7
vegetables, legumes	4	4-5	5-9
fruit	2	1-2	3-4
milk, yogurt, cheese	3	3	3-5
meat, fish, poultry, eggs, nuts, legumes	½-1	1-1½	11
extra foods	1-2	1-2	1-3

what's a serving?

Grains and cereals 2 slices of bread; 1 medium bread roll; 1 cup cooked rice or pasta noodles; 1 cup porridge; 1⅓ cup breakfast cereal flakes or ½ cup muesli.

Vegetables and legumes ½ cup cooked vegetables, dried peas, beans or lentils; 1 cup salad vegetables; 1 potato.

Fruit 1 medium piece e.g. apple, banana, orange, pear; 2 small pieces e.g. apricots, kiwifruit, plums; 1 cup canned fruit; ½ cup juice; 4 dried apricots; 1½ tablespoons sultanas.

Milk, yogurt, cheese 1 cup milk; ½ cup evaporated milk; 2 slices cheese; ¾ cup yogurt; 1 cup custard.

Meat, fish, poultry, eggs, nuts, legumes 65-100g cooked meat or chicken e.g. ½ cup lean mince, 2 small chops or 2 slices roast meat; ½ cup cooked beans, lentils, chickpeas etc; 1 cooked small fish fillet (80-120g); 3 fish fingers; a small can of tuna or salmon; 4 prawns; 2 small eggs; ⅓ cup peanuts or almonds; ¼ cup seeds.

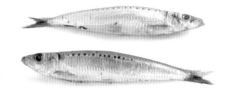

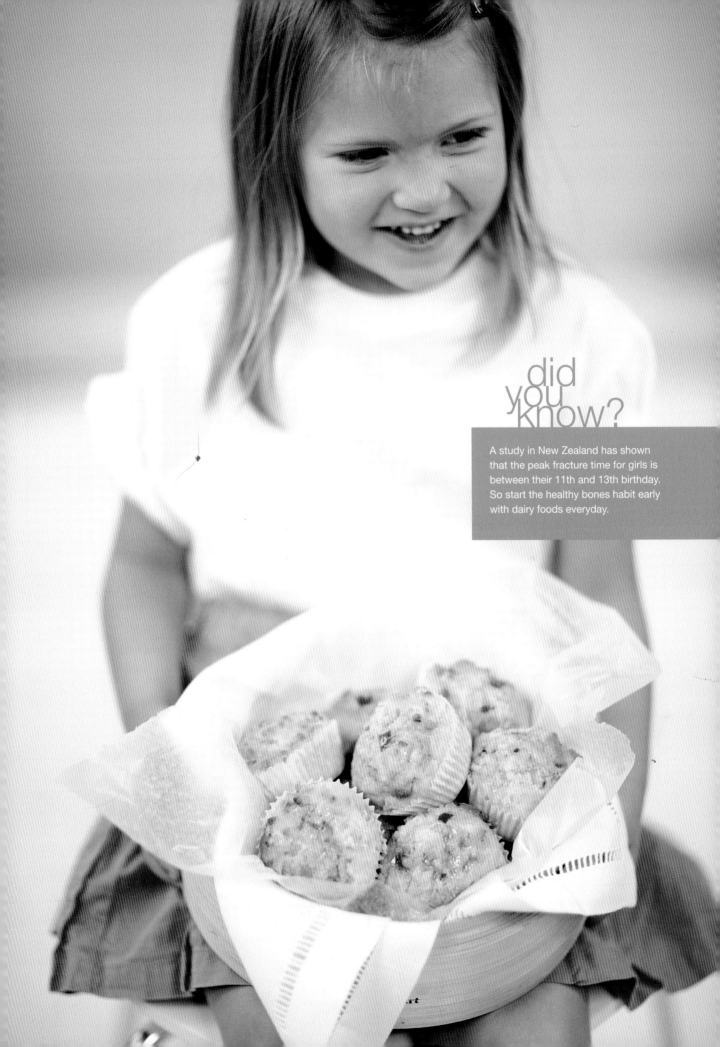

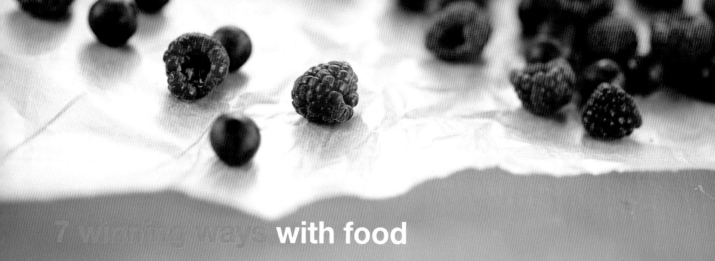

7 winning ways **with food**

With so much information about food and nutrition it sometimes feels like you need a nutrition degree to sort through what's best for your family when, in fact, the answers are often found in getting the basics right. If you focus on these seven winning ways with food, you're well on your way to growing a happy, healthy child.

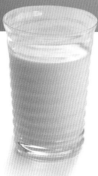

foods for strong bones and teeth

Get enough calcium intake everyday from:
- Milk on cereal or to drink
- Yogurt or yogurt drinks
- Calcium-boosted orange juice
- Cheese as a snack, in sandwiches and in cooking
- Smoothies with milk and yogurt
- Canned fish with bones
- Calcium-fortified soy drinks

antioxidants

Antioxidants occur naturally in the body. They mop up excess free radicals before they can do any harm. Free radicals are a normal product of metabolism (processes occurring within the body's cells that are necessary for life). However, an excess of free radicals can attack healthy cells, damage healthy DNA and weaken the immune system. To slow down the affects of free radicals, it is important to eat plenty of fresh foods that are full of antioxidants.

1 role model healthy behaviours

The foundations of healthy eating in your children come from you as parents. It makes sense that kids will naturally mimic the eating and lifestyle behaviours of their parents. Not only are you their provider, but you're also their biggest role models. And research is proving the amazing strength parents play in being positive role models. So, if you're skipping breakfast, can you expect them to want to sit and eat alone? If you're drinking soft drinks with meals, can you really expect them not to ask for one, too, and stick to water? If mum and dad are eating takeaways, should you really expect your preschoolers to sit and eat their vegies?

The best approach is to look at a healthy-lifestyle plan for the whole family that starts from the top down, and not have different foods or rules for the kids. When mums and dads role model healthy eating and physical activity behaviours, often the kids simply come along for the ride. That's what they love to do: spend time with, and participate in, what their parents do. The best place for kids to learn healthy-eating behaviour is with family meals. You may not be able to sit down together every night of the week, but try as many times as you can. And try brunch together on Sundays, too.

2 keep it real, keep it whole

Another winning way is to get back to basics with whole foods. Choose foods close to the source and in their natural state, like fresh fruits, pulses, vegetables, wholegrains, lean meats, fish, eggs and dairy; you're certain to get foods naturally brimming in nutrients. These foods tend to be high in nutrients, but not high in kilojoules as they do not have added fat or sugar. These foods help your child grow, but also gives them shiny hair, clear skin, strong nails and sparkling teeth. So try and base much of your child's food intake around these whole foods. Encourage them to eat foods like apples with skin to boost their fibre and antioxidant intake, probiotic yogurts with active cultures, fish without crumbed coatings and wholegrains.

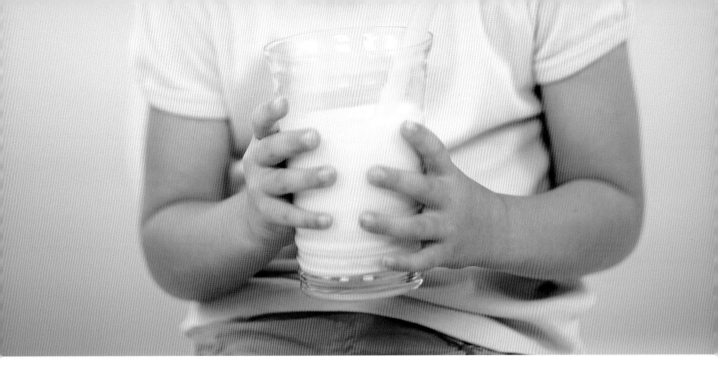

Wholegrains refer to grain-based foods that use all three layers of the grain – the bran (the outer layer), endosperm (the main part) and germ (the smallest part). And it's in these three layers that optimal nutrients and antioxidants are found. Good choices include oats, untoasted muesli, wholegrain breakfast cereals, brown rice and mixed-grain breads.

3 eat rainbows

This is a clever extension of the food-variety principle and another winning way to encourage your kids to eat a varied diet. All you need to do is follow the song *I Can Sing a Rainbow*, and go for red and yellow and pink and green, purple and orange and blue. When you eat a rainbow, especially with plant foods, you consume foods from a wide spectrum of colours that maximise nutrients and protective components. Plant foods contain special components called bioactives, which act as antioxidants and play other important roles in the body. There's lycopene in red-pigmented foods like tomatoes, lutein from gold kiwifruit and anthocyanins, found in blueberries, just to name a few. The idea is to make each meal and snack as colourful as possible to reap these plant rewards.

foods for energy

Energise those muscles and brain cells with **nutritious carbohydrates like:**
• Wholegrains such as oats, wheat, barley, rye, rice, triticale, buckwheat, quinoa and corn
• Wholegrain breakfast cereals
• Wholegrain breads and muffins
• Fruit (fresh, stewed, dried)
• Starchy vegetables like potato, kumara, peas, corn and pumpkin
• Pasta, noodles and rice

Iron-rich foods like:
• Lean red meat
• Liver and kidney
• Dark meat of poultry
• Green leafy vegetables like spinach, silver beet, broccoli and asian greens*
• Legumes*

(*needs foods rich in vitamin C to help absorption)

instead of	try
canned peaches for dessert	adding some strawberries and kiwifruit
meat and two veg	going for more stir-fries and pasta dishes with a number of different vegetables
plain cereal for breakfast	adding some tropical fruit salad on top
ham sandwich for lunch	adding some tomato slices and grated carrot
green salad with dinner	making a rainbow salad with red tomato, yellow capsicum, purple cabbage and char-grilled kumara

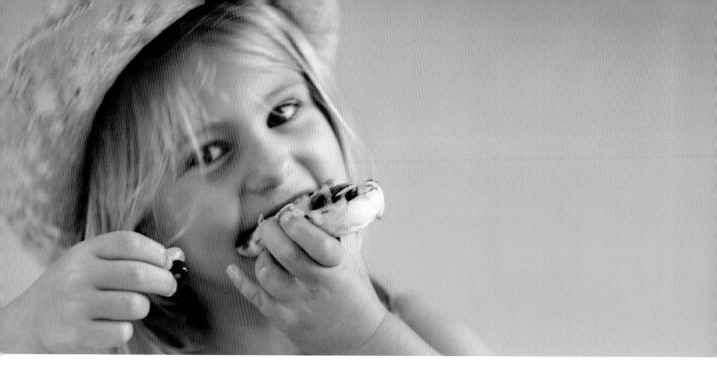

4 go for friendly fats

Everyone needs a little daily fat to function properly. Fat is an energy source and is necessary to make hormone-like compounds that regulate body processes. Fat also acts as a carrier for the fat-soluble vitamins, A, D, E and K. The dietary guidelines for children and adolescents say care should be taken to limit saturated fat and moderate total-fat intake. So the key is to get a little friendly fats each day and limit the rest.

• Friendly polyunsaturated fats: vegetable oils and margarines and certain nuts and seeds.
• Friendly monounsaturated fats: olive, sunola and canola oil, avocado and certain nuts.
• Friendly omega-3 fats: fish oils found in deep-sea fish especially sardines, tuna, salmon, mackerel and herring, canola oil, walnuts and linseeds.
• Friendly omega-6 fats: nuts and seeds and their oils.

5 snack smart

Kids have little tummies and big energy needs, so regular mid-meal snacks are vital. While unhealthy snacking has been partially blamed for the obesity epidemic, the right snacks can boost energy and concentration at school, and help meet nutrient requirements. Snack smart on the following foods:

• Fresh fruit
• Yogurt
• Low-fat grain-and-fruit based bars
• Mugs of homemade soup
• Snack-size cans of baked beans
• Fruit snack packs
• Small servings of dried fruit and nuts
• Homemade fruit bread and mini muffins

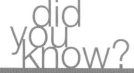

did you know?

Vitamin D boosts bone health as it helps the body better absorb calcium. Dairy foods or breakfast cereals with added vitamin D can help kids reach their peak growth.

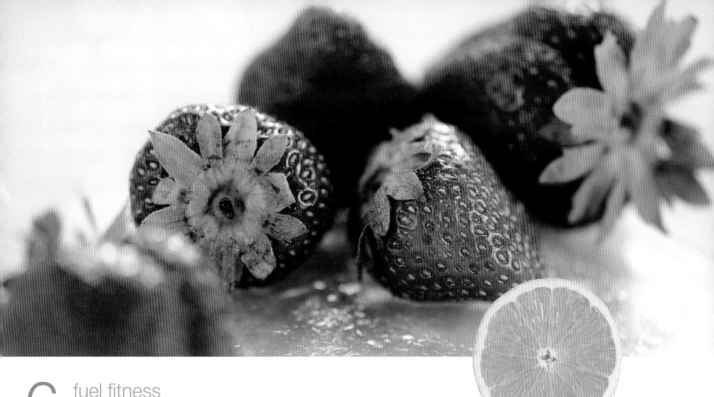

6 fuel fitness

Carbohydrates are the key fuel for our bodies and vital to fuel fitness. In order to be active, kids need a steady supply of carbohydrates to keep their engines running. When foods containing carbohydrates are digested, they are broken down into glucose in the bloodstream. The glucose can either be used immediately for energy or, if not required, stored in the muscle as glycogen, to be used later. Just remember, more is not necessarily better. Your child's body can only store a limited amount as glycogen, any excess carbohydrates will be stored as body fat.

Aim to ensure all meals contain some energy-giving carbohydrates like breakfast cereal topped with fruit, sandwiches for lunch, and rice, pasta or noodles with dinner.

Very active kids may need some extra servings of carbohydrates, and especially a high-carbohydrate recovery snack as soon as possible after a strenuous training session. Good choices for a fast refuel include a smoothie or drinking yogurt.

7 add the fun factor

While you don't need to become a qualified children's entertainer or turn every meal into a party, there's a lot to be said about putting the fun factor into food. Food is so much more than simple nourishment. It's a fundamental part of our social life, our celebrations and traditions. Aim to instil a positive relationship with food in your kids, and keep things fun. This can be as simple as serving up a smoothie with a curly straw or in a brightly coloured glass with an umbrella. Or try having some sushi or a fish and chip meal at the beach along with some active beach kick and run fun. You'll find more fun factor ideas in *getting your kids involved* (see page 19).

foods for clear skin

The latest research on diet and acne prevention is pointing to a limit on the amount of processed foods like sugary breakfast cereals, soft drinks, takeaway foods, cakes and biscuits, and an eating plan based on:

Lower GI carbohydrates like:
• Pasta and basmati rice
• Wholegrain breads and breakfast cereals
• Orchard fruits, such as apples, oranges, peaches and pears
• Yogurt

Protein-rich foods at every meal like:
• Lean beef, lamb or veal 3-4 times a week and fish twice a week
• Legumes like baked beans, lentils and chickpeas
• Eggs
• Reduced-fat dairy foods

Monounsaturated fats like:
• Canola and olive oil
• Avocado
• Nuts and seeds

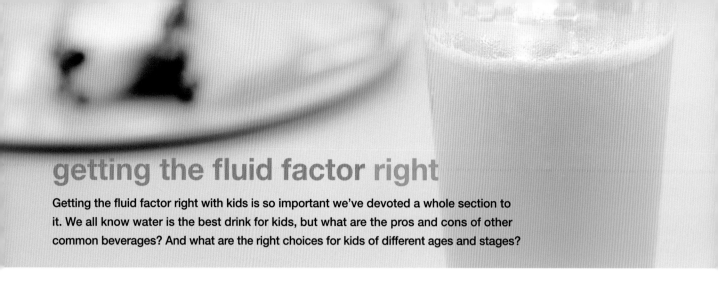

getting the fluid factor right

Getting the fluid factor right with kids is so important we've devoted a whole section to it. We all know water is the best drink for kids, but what are the pros and cons of other common beverages? And what are the right choices for kids of different ages and stages?

top tip A great family habit is to always have a jug of iced water on the dinner table. You might like to spritz it up with some lemon, lime or orange slices.

top tip Make sure you dilute all juice with two-thirds water for younger children and limit this to one glass per day.

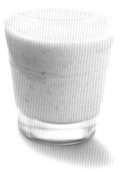

top tip Get older kids and teens to keep the milk drinking habit by serving up an icy cold breakfast smoothie.

water

Water is essential to life, and the best all-round hydrator. Although we do not have fluid recommendations for children, the best advice is to use thirst as a good indicator of fluid needs. Children should drink to quench thirst and then a little more. Water is the "number one" drink for all kids, and should be the only fluid that makes its way into drink bottles. Encourage your kids to drink regularly from the bubblers or fountains at school, especially during hot weather. Sports drinks can be useful for active children who play sport (see *sports and energy drinks*, page 15).

fruit juice

This is where the debate starts to get juicy. Juicing has generally been given a healthy and herbal image, but juices are not necessarily the best regular beverage choice for kids, or adults for that matter. With juices you're getting such a concentrated source of fruit sugars and kilojoules, as several pieces of whole fruit are used to make one glass. This means juices can add loads of extra kilojoules to your day, and do not have the same amount of fibre, or the fullness factor, as the equivalent pieces of fruit. A daily juice can be a good way of helping older kids and teens reach their fruit and vegetable target. However, there are particular concerns with young children and juice. These centre on the connection with tooth decay, as well as high juice consumption causing inadequate food intakes. So called "juice-aholics" are common in the toddler years where kids graze on fruit juice all day and lose their appetite for meals.

milk

Milk should be the second drink of choice for kids. Young children have the milk drinking habit, but this tends to drop off as they age, and by the teen years many, especially girls, unfortunately steer clear of milk. Milk is one of the most readily available and absorbable sources of calcium, plus it's packed with other essential nutrients like riboflavin and protein. However, it also contains saturated fat, and for this reason, the Dietary Guidelines for Children and Adolescents now recommend reduced-fat varieties of milk for any child over the age of two years.

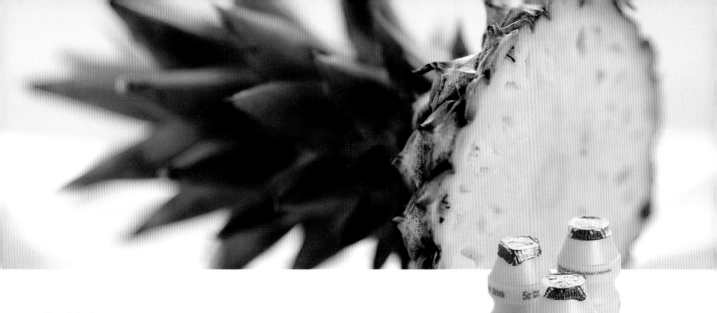

soft drinks

We now have alarming research on the soft drink consumption habits of Aussie kids and evidence of the links with overweight and obesity. Recent research has shown that 78 per cent of all 12-17 year old children had consumed soft drink in the week preceding the survey, and the latest national nutrition survey found that around half of all teenagers and over 25 per cent of 2-3 year old children had consumed soft drink during the previous 24 hours. Teenage boys aged 16-18 drink an average of 840ml per day, double the intake of teenage girls.

Despite their marketing hype, soft drinks have little going for them in the nutrition stakes. You're getting nothing apart from flavours, colours, a few bubbles and loads of sugar. According to recent research there is a 60 per cent increased risk of children becoming overweight with each additional can or glass of soft drink consumed each day. These concerns over soft drinks and the obesity problem have led to their recent ban in many Aussie schools.

sports and energy drinks

These drinks are often lumped together, but they have very different formulations and uses.

Sports drinks are designed to maximise hydration, during or after strenuous sport or physical activity. They contain just the right amount of carbohydrate and electrolytes an active body needs. But the emphasis must be on "active bodies". Children involved in competition sport or long distance endurance events can benefit from sports drinks as part of their training and competition diet. But remind your older kids that a walk to the local milk bar and back doesn't warrant a sports drink in return.

Energy drinks, as their name implies, claim to give you energy. But this is simply from a big hit of caffeine either as a caffeine additive or guarana (a stimulant derived from the seeds of a Brazilian plant of the same name). Their effect is no different than a double-shot espresso, and caution should certainly be taken with kids and caffeine.

top tip If your teens go for a regular soft drink fix, try and get them to alternate it with a fruit smoothie, milkshake or drinking yogurt for valuable nutrients. And, if weight is an issue, encourage them to switch to a diet alternative to their favourite soft drink and then only for special occasions.

top tip Talk to your child's coach about their opinion of sports drinks and how best to use them for their type of sport.

did you know?

Drinking yogurts are not that common with kids, but they are a nutrition winner. Not only are they cool and refreshing, calcium-charged and protein-packed, but they're also full of probiotic bacteria to boost immunity.

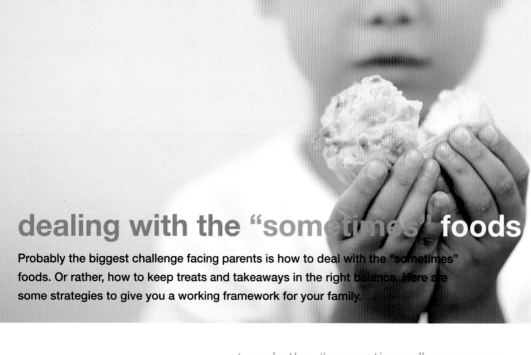

dealing with the "sometimes" foods

Probably the biggest challenge facing parents is how to deal with the "sometimes" foods. Or rather, how to keep treats and takeaways in the right balance. Here are some strategies to give you a working framework for your family.

teach the "sometimes" message

A good strategy is to talk to your children about everyday and sometimes foods, rather than good and bad foods. All food has a place in a healthy diet, it's just the frequency and quantity that counts. It's likely that everyday foods in your family include wholegrain breads and cereals, fruits and vegetables, dairy foods, and so on, and sometimes foods will be things like chocolates, lollies, ice-creams, chips and cake. But different families will have their own individual lists.

decide together on treat times

Children have an innate preference for sweetness and love the bright colours, wrappings and advertising of popular treat foods. Research shows that completely depriving children of treat-type foods only fuels their desire, so they end up going for it at parties and other all-you-can-eat opportunities. But how do you get the balance right? Rather than go into constant battle in the confectionery aisle at the supermarket or when packing the lunchbox each morning, sit down and decide together on treat times. Parents are often surprised at how even young kids can grasp family guidelines on foods. You may decide together that treat time is once or twice a week after school and stop for an ice-block or portion-controlled chocolate on the walk home. Or perhaps you allow a once-a-week lunch order or treat from the school canteen. Families will differ in their approaches, but the key for all is consistency. Decide together on the treat times and don't budge, no matter how much your kids pester.

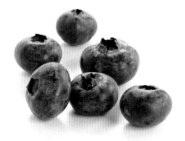

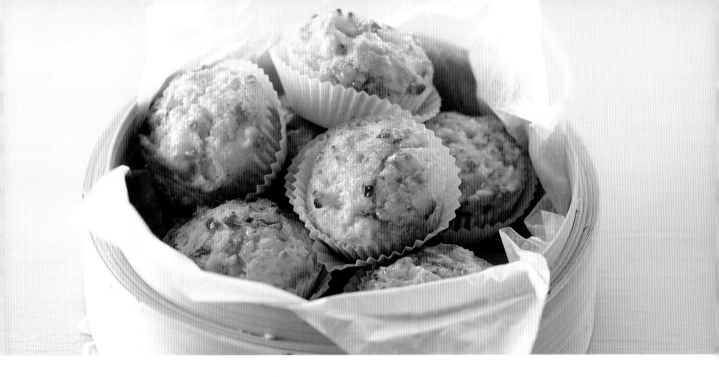

keep treats in their place

The old saying "out of sight out of mind" certainly applies to kids. When you keep
plenty of everyday foods and snacks on hand, your kids will go for these first. So
keep the fruit bowl filled, stock the fridge with snack-sized yogurts and keep grain-
based bars, wholegrain biscuits or air-popped popcorn in snack-sized portions.
Likewise, make sure your treat foods are put away on the high shelf in the pantry.
Better still, keep an opaque box for treats, so they can't be seen every time the
pantry door is opened. Also think twice about treats in the lunchbox. Today, kids
bring a huge range of different foods to school but, rest assured, the snack pack
of chips gets eaten before the sandwich.

slot in a regular takeaway

As well as giving mums and dads a break, takeaway night is usually a big highlight
for kids. But it's easy to fall into the trap of "I'm too tired to cook" and end up having
one too many takeaways or one too many visits to the local fast-food restaurant.

A smart strategy is to slot in a regular night either once a week, or fortnight, and
stick the rest of the time to the fabulous family-friendly recipes in this book. Make
sure you also aim to increase the variety with takeaways rather than going for the
one type each time. Have your kids try healthier picks from Thai, Japanese, Italian
and Chinese takeaway food, as well as the old favourites, pizza and fish and chips.

kitchen capers

Your kids can learn so much about food and nutrition just being involved in your daily
food shopping, preparation, cooking and family meals. However, getting kids in the
kitchen is a little daunting for many parents. It's hard enough just pulling a family meal
together in lightning speed, without an extra pair of little hands wanting to help. While
no one likes mess, it's best not to be too fastidious about cleanliness when it comes
to kids in the kitchen. You'll be right if you stick to our kid-friendly recipes.

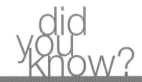

Some takeaways with a healthy image
can still be laden with fat, salt and sugar.
Next time you take out a salad, noodles
or wrap, ask if you can also take away
their nutrition leaflet to check out the
counts. Some fast-food chains are even
putting the stats on the wrap with a full
nutrition information panel.

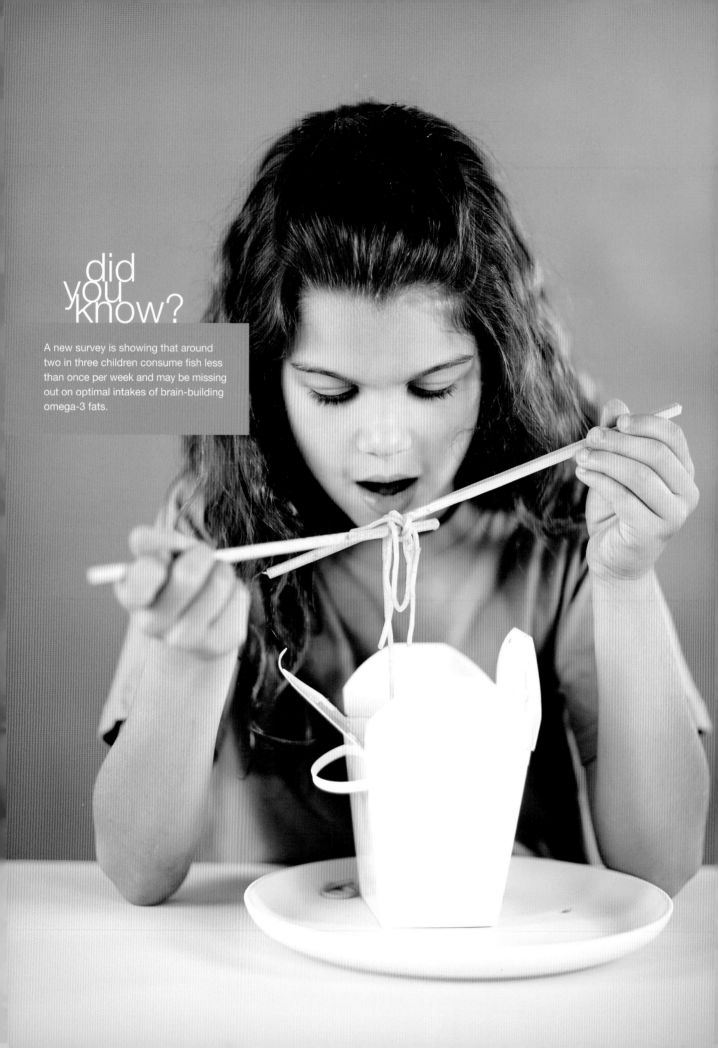

did you know?

A new survey is showing that around two in three children consume fish less than once per week and may be missing out on optimal intakes of brain-building omega-3 fats.

getting your kids involved

if you're unsure about	smart solution
finding the time to cook together	try making muffins or pancakes for a leisurely Sunday brunch when the pressure's off from the mid week.
teaching your kids where food comes from	grow a herb or cherry tomato pot together; go strawberry picking or visit a farmers' or fish market.
encouraging your teens that cooking is cool	watch a celebrity chef cooking show together and try a sample recipe.
a sleepover solution that caters to all tastes	make your own pizzas from pita bread and a selection of toppings.
the safety aspects of young kids in the kitchen	start them off with a plastic picnic knife slicing soft fruit, or helping to stir cake mixture rather than stovetop cooking.
getting your kids to increase the variety of their meals	get them to decorate and keep individual recipe books where they can list their food preferences and favourite dishes.
dragging your kids around the supermarket	set them some fun detective tasks as you go down the aisles. Who can find dry biscuits with wholegrains? Who can spot a vegetable beginning with "B"?
ways to make fruit fun	allow a little play time and make fruit faces together at snack time – try blueberry eyes, watermelon smiles, kiwifruit cheeks and star fruit hair. Or try threading fruit kebabs.
encouraging them to try a new dish	have a cuisine theme night where you try Spanish, Mexican, Italian or Japanese. Set the table to your theme, play some appropriate music and talk about different cultures and eating styles.
getting young kids to stay at the table	move it outside on a balmy evening and eat picnic style at a local park or in the backyard.

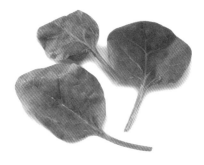

foods for an immunity boost

Boost your child's defences with plenty of:
• Probiotic yogurt
• Vitamin C from citrus fruits, kiwifruit, tomatoes and red capsicum
• Iron from lean red meat, pâté, green leafy vegetables and fortified breakfast cereal
• Zinc from lean red meat, seafood, legumes* and fortified-breakfast cereals* (*needs animal protein to help absorption)

grow well

Just like the plants in your garden, the little ones in your life need some nurturing and extra care from time to time. From the age of 10, your little sprouts start their growth spurts and it's a good idea to keep check on their intake of the important growth nutrients like calcium, iron and zinc. Among their other roles in the body, calcium is needed for bone building, zinc is needed for tissue repair and development and iron is needed for the formation of haemoglobin and red blood cells. Requirements differ by age and gender, but on average your child should be aiming for at least three serves of dairy foods a day for calcium; 9-12mg a day of zinc; and 6-8mg of iron for under 12 years, and 10-13mg of iron for 12-15 year olds. To give you an idea of how to clock up iron and zinc we've included these handy food counters.

zinc counter

which food?	what's a serving?	how much zinc (mg)?
almonds	25 pieces	1.0
apricots, dried	½ cup	0.6
beans, baked, canned	1 cup	1.4
beef, lean, cooked	100g	5.3
bread, wholemeal	1 slice	0.3
breakfast cereal, fortified	1 cup	1.1
broccoli, boiled	1 piece	0.3
cheese, reduced-fat	30g	1.5
chicken, lean, cooked	100g	1.2
chickpeas, canned	1 cup	1.7
egg, boiled	1 egg	0.5
fish, steamed	100g	0.7
kidney, cooked	100g	3.0
lamb, lean, cooked	100g	4.3
milk, reduced-fat	1 cup	1.0
muesli, natural	1 cup	2.1
oats, rolled, cooked	1 cup	0.8
oysters, raw	6 oysters	59
pasta, wholemeal, cooked	1 cup	0.9
peanuts	30g	0.9
pork, lean, cooked	100g	3.0
rice, brown, cooked	1 cup	1.6
seeds, pumpkin, sunflower	30g	1.9
sesame seeds	30g	1.7
spinach, cooked	1 cup	0.9
tuna, canned	100g	0.9
vita brits	2 biscuits	0.4
walnuts	30g	0.8
weeties	1 cup	0.5

iron counter

which food?	what's a serving?	how much iron (mg)?
almonds	25 pieces	1.1
apricots, dried	½ cup	2.1
beans, baked, canned	1 cup	4.4
beef, lean, cooked	100g	3.1
bread, wholemeal	1 slice	0.5
breakfast cereal, fortified	1 cup	6.7
broccoli, boiled	1 piece	0.4
cheese, reduced-fat	30g	0.7
chicken, lean, cooked	100g	3.1
chickpeas, canned	1 cup	1.7
egg, boiled	1 egg	0.9
fish, steamed	100g	0.7
lamb, lean, cooked	100g	2.4
muesli, natural	1 cup	4.7
oats, rolled, cooked	1 cup	1.8
oysters, raw	6 oysters	3.5
pasta, wholemeal, cooked	1 cup	2.7
pâté	1 tablespoon	1.5
peanuts	30g	0.7
pork, lean, cooked	100g	1.2
rice, brown, cooked	1 cup	0.9
salmon, canned	100g	1.5
seeds, pumpkin	30g	3.0
sesame seeds	30g	1.6
spinach, cooked	1 cup	4.4
tuna, canned	100g	1.0
vita brits	2 biscuits	2.6
walnuts	30g	0.8
weeties	1 cup	0.9

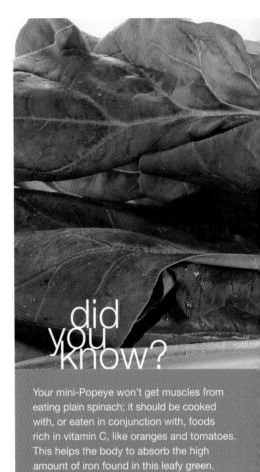

did you know?

Your mini-Popeye won't get muscles from eating plain spinach; it should be cooked with, or eaten in conjunction with, foods rich in vitamin C, like oranges and tomatoes. This helps the body to absorb the high amount of iron found in this leafy green.

a day in the life...

The following meal plans give you an idea of the types and amounts of foods required to achieve a nutritionally-balanced intake for your child. While there are no actual fluid requirements for children, the health message for a 5 year old is to drink at least ½ glass (125ml) of water per meal and according to thirst during the day; a 10 year old should drink at least a full glass (250ml) of water per meal and according to thirst during the day.

a day in the life of a 5 year old	
morning rush	1 serving rhubarb, muesli and yogurt cups (p32); ½ glass of reduced-fat milk (125ml)
in the lunchbox	1 egg salad sandwich (p44); bunch of grapes; 1 piece fruit muesli slice (p101); water bottle
after school fix	1 serving strawberry soy smoothie (p42)
early dinner and off to bed	½ serving minty lamb cutlets with mixed vegie smash (p71); ¼ serving large pesto corn cobs (p78); ½ glass (125ml) water; 1 orange crème caramel (p88)
nutritional analysis per day	7045kJ (1700 cal); 57g total fat (19g saturated fat); 219g carbohydrate; 63g protein; 18g fibre; 845mg calcium; 10mg iron; 7mg zinc

a day in the life of a 10 year old	
big breakfast	1 serving baked beans, bacon, tomato and chives (p35); 1 serving carrot, orange and ginger juice (p41)
in the lunchbox	1 serving mediterranean tuna baguette (p45); 1 slice banana loaf (p102); 1 apple
hunger buster before sport	1 cream cheese, corn and sweet chilli muffin (p109); 1 glass reduced-fat milk (250ml)
family dinner	2 beef enchiladas (p56); ½ serving tomato and capsicum salad (p76); 1 serving fruit salad and yogurt trifle (p92); 1 glass water (250ml) with lemon slices
nutritional analysis per day	9405kJ (2240 cal); 72g total fat (25g saturated fat); 271g carbohydrate; 108g protein; 33g fibre; 1216mg calcium; 14mg iron; 13mg zinc

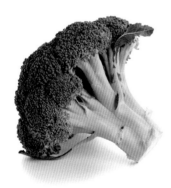

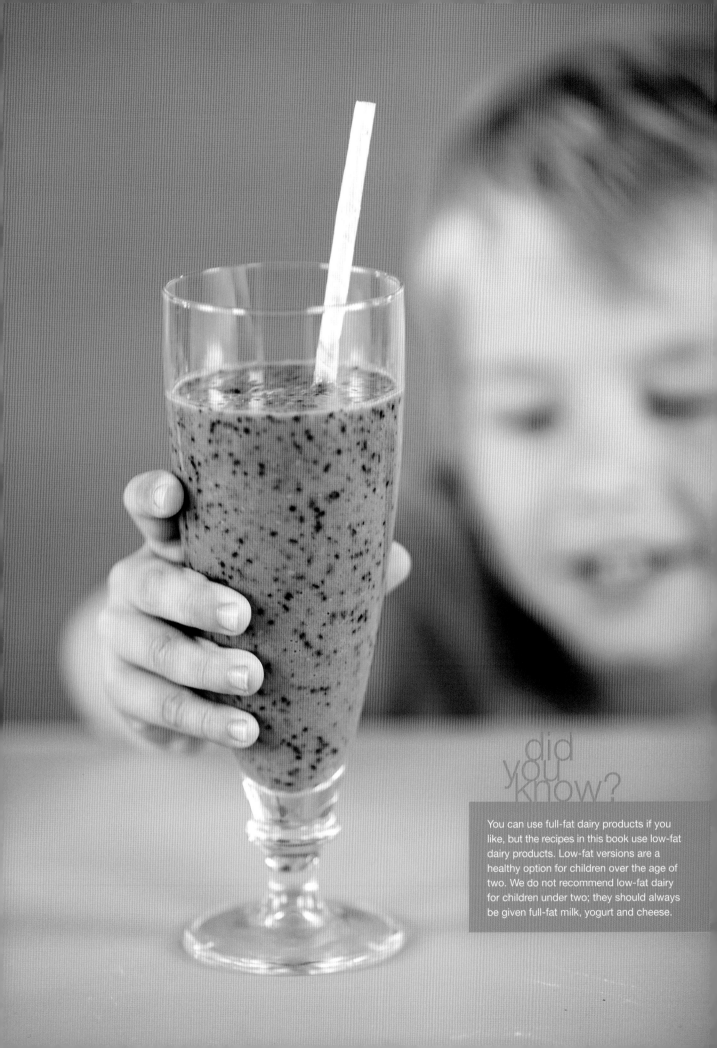

breakfasts

apple and raisin french toast

preparation time 20 minutes
(plus cooling time)
cooking time 15 minutes **serves** 4
per serving 10.3g total fat
(4.3g saturated fat); 1668kJ
(399 cal); 60.6g carbohydrate;
13.6g protein; 3.5g fibre

*Here, french toast gets a whole new
look, and it's bound to be a hit with
young and old alike.*

1 large apple (200g), peeled,
  cored, sliced thinly
2 tablespoons water
¼ cup (35g) coarsely
  chopped raisins
½ loaf unsliced white bread (320g)
3 eggs
½ cup (125ml) low-fat milk
1 tablespoon honey
½ teaspoon finely grated
  orange rind
½ teaspoon ground cinnamon
20g butter
2 tablespoons icing sugar

1 Place apple and the water in small saucepan; bring to a boil. Reduce heat; simmer, covered, about 5 minutes or until apple is just tender. Remove from heat; stir in raisins. Cool 15 minutes.
2 Meanwhile, slice bread into quarters; cut each piece three-quarters of the way through. Divide apple mixture among bread pockets.
3 Whisk eggs in medium bowl; whisk in milk, honey, rind and cinnamon.
4 Heat half the butter in large frying pan. Dip two bread pockets into egg mixture, one at a time; cook, uncovered, until browned both sides.
5 Remove from pan; cover to keep warm. Repeat with remaining butter and bread. Cut pockets into quarters; serve sprinkled with sifted icing sugar.

did you know? Breakfast is the most important meal of the day as it breaks the overnight fast. Research shows that kids who eat breakfast are more likely to meet nutrient requirements, keep a healthy weight and perform better physically and cognitively at school.

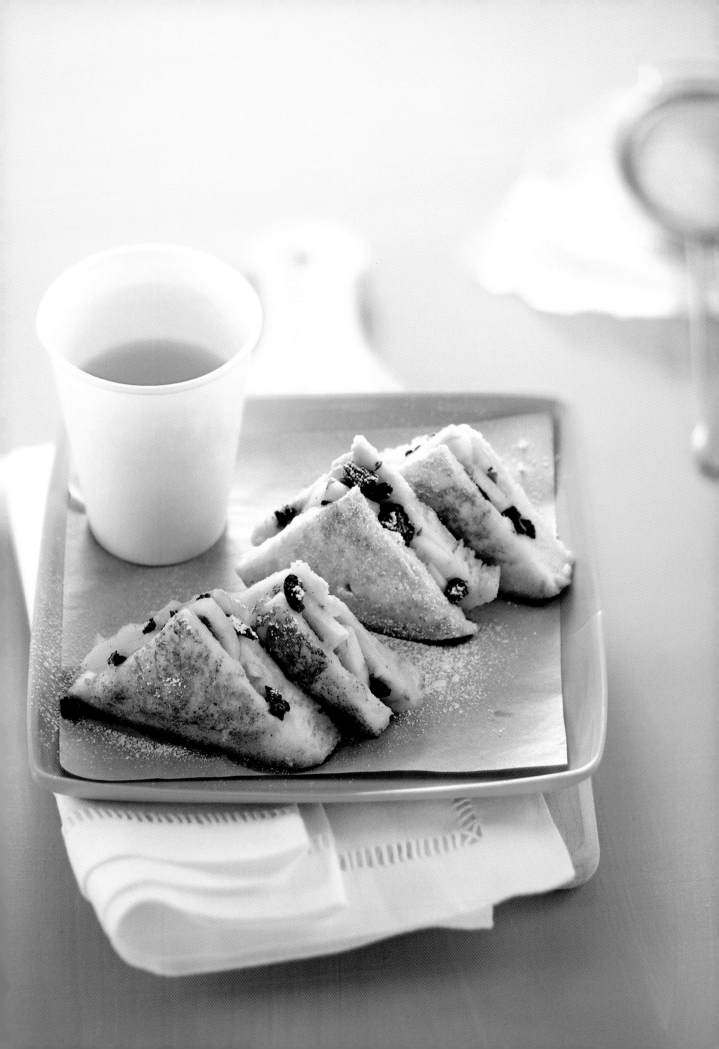

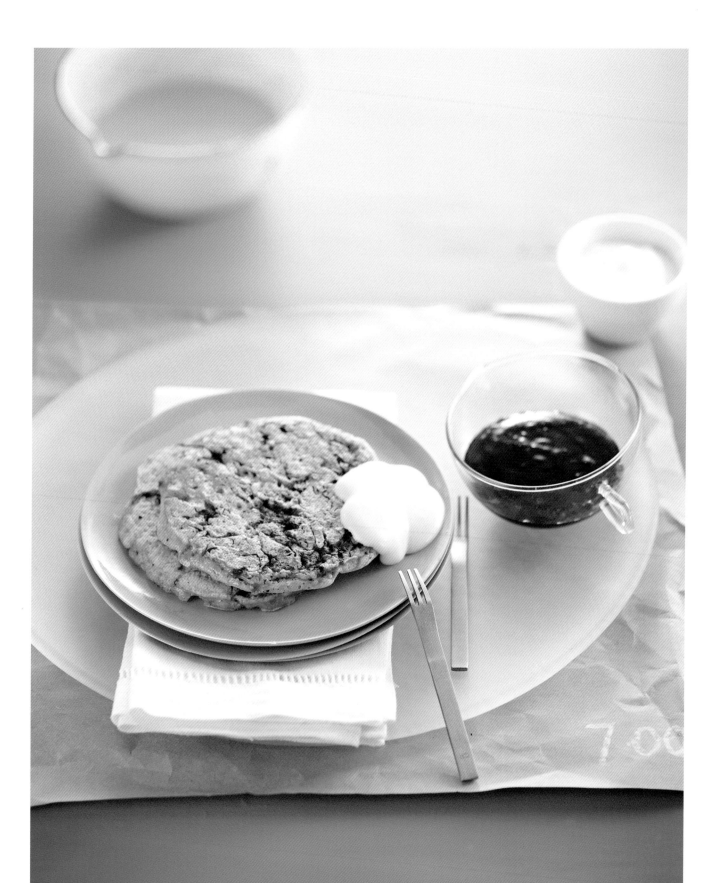

berry
buckwheat
pancakes

preparation time 10 minutes
(plus refrigeration time)
cooking time 10 minutes **makes** 8
per pancake 2g total fat
(0.6g saturated fat); 786kJ
(188 cal); 33.7g carbohydrate;
7.6g protein; 1.5g fibre

*Pretty as a picture with their berry
swirls, any leftover pancakes can be
taken to school for a morning-tea treat.
You can find buckwheat flour at health
food stores.*

1 cup (150g) self-raising flour
⅔ cup (100g) buckwheat flour
2 tablespoons caster sugar
½ teaspoon ground cinnamon
2 eggs, beaten lightly
1½ cups (375ml) low-fat milk
1 cup (150g) frozen
   mixed berries, thawed
2 tablespoons orange juice
2 tablespoons icing sugar

1 Combine flours, caster sugar and
cinnamon in medium bowl; gradually
whisk in combined egg and milk until
batter is smooth. Cover; refrigerate
30 minutes.

2 Meanwhile, blend or process
berries, juice and icing sugar
until pureed.

3 Pour ⅓ cup batter into heated
oiled medium frying pan. Spoon
1 level teaspoon puree on top of
pancake batter; using skewer, gently
swirl puree through batter to marble.
Cook pancake, uncovered, until
bubbles begin to appear on surface.
Turn pancake; cook until firm.

4 Repeat process, using ⅓ cup
batter and 1 teaspoon puree for
each pancake, to make a total of
eight pancakes.

5 Serve pancakes with remaining
berry puree, and low-fat yogurt, if
you like.

cheesy scrambled eggs with spinach

preparation time 5 minutes
cooking time 5 minutes **serves** 4
per serving 13.8g total fat
(5.4g saturated fat); 790kJ
(189 cal); 1g carbohydrate;
15.3g protein; 0.3g fibre

A fantastic fuel-boost to start your family's day, these are the most delicious eggs you'll ever taste.

8 eggs
⅓ cup (80g) reduced-fat
   spreadable cream cheese
50g baby spinach leaves,
   chopped coarsely

1 Whisk eggs in medium bowl until combined then whisk in cheese and spinach.
2 Cook mixture, stirring gently, in heated oiled large frying pan over low heat until almost set. Serve with wholemeal toast, if you like.

did you know? Eggs are a nutritional powerhouse providing 18 different vitamins and minerals, high-quality protein and important antioxidants. They make a great protein serve at breakfast for growing kids.

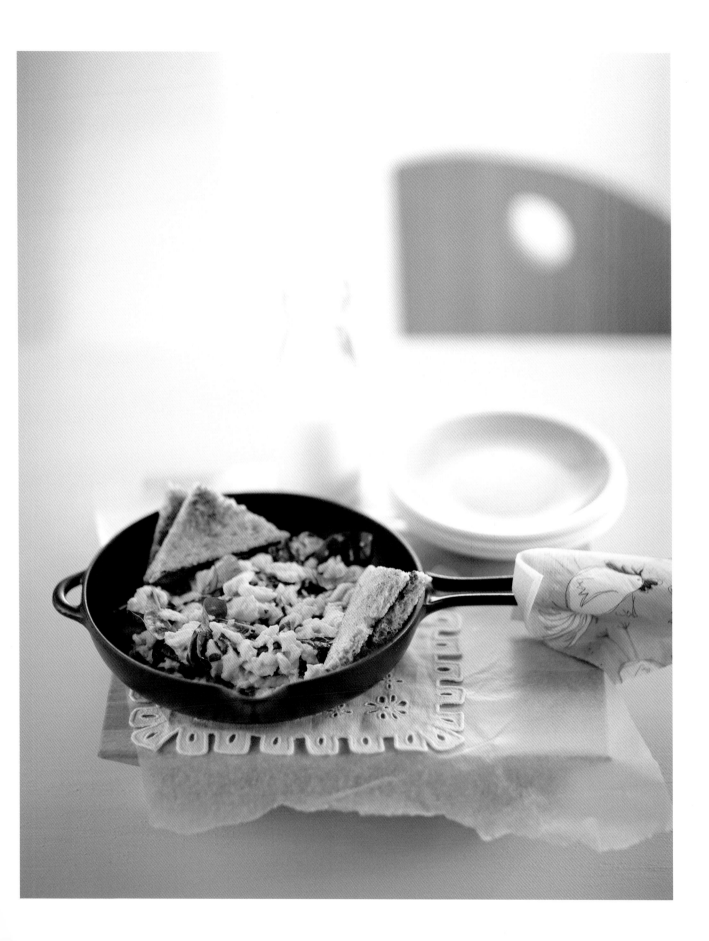

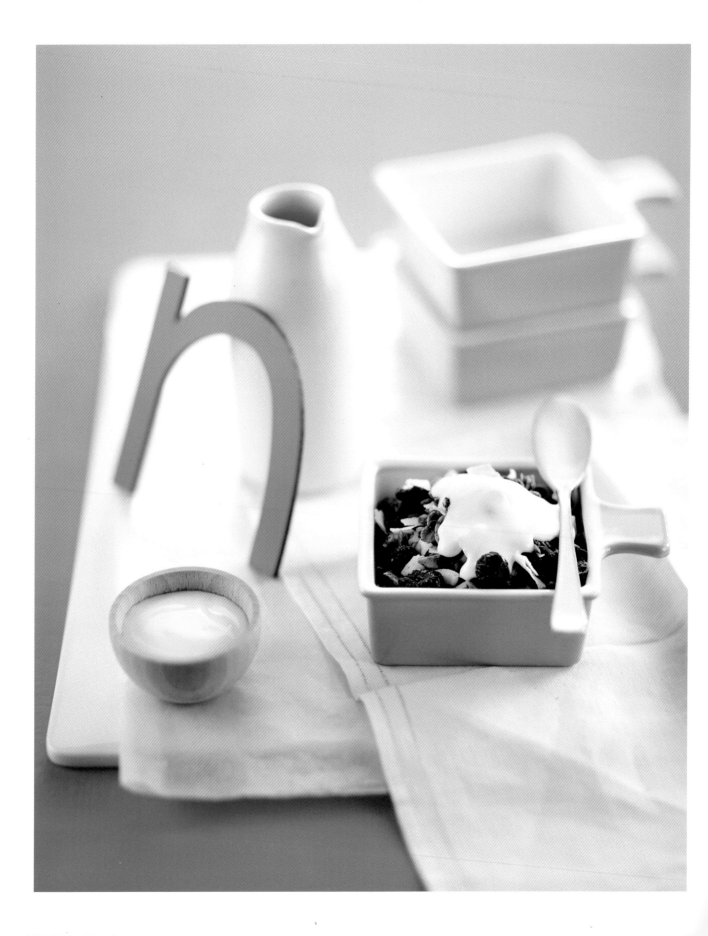

cranberry and almond granola

preparation time 5 minutes
cooking time 40 minutes **makes** 5 cups
per ½ cup 12.7g total fat
(1.9g saturated fat); 1062kJ
(254 cal); 29.1g carbohydrate;
4.4g protein; 3.2g fibre
tip You can double or triple the
quantities shown here, and store
granola in an airtight container in the
refrigerator for up to three months.

*Once you've tried this homemade
granola, you'll never go back to
store-bought again. We recommend
a serving size of ½ cup.*

½ cup (125ml) cranberry juice
⅓ cup (75g) firmly packed
   brown sugar
1 tablespoon vegetable oil
2 cups (180g) rolled oats
½ cup (70g) slivered almonds
½ cup (60g) coarsely chopped
   roasted pecans
1 teaspoon ground cinnamon
⅓ cup (15g) flaked coconut
1 cup (130g) craisins

1 Preheat oven to 180°C/160°C
fan-forced.
2 Combine juice, sugar and oil in
small saucepan; stir over low heat
until sugar dissolves.
3 Meanwhile, combine oats, nuts
and cinnamon in large bowl. Stir
in juice mixture. Spread mixture
evenly over two oven trays. Cook,
uncovered, 30 minutes, stirring
occasionally. Stir coconut and
craisins into oat mixture. Cook,
uncovered, 5 minutes.
4 Remove trays from oven; cool
granola on trays. Serve with milk
or yogurt, if you like.

did you know? A native of North America, cranberries have a distinct
sweet-tart taste. They were a staple food of the American Indians who were
accustomed to eating them fresh or dried (forebears of today's craisins).
The Indians recognised their health and nutrition benefits, using them in
traditional medicine and to supplement their diet during long, cold winters.

rhubarb, muesli and yogurt cups

preparation time 10 minutes
(plus refrigeration time)
cooking time 10 minutes serves 4
per serving 1.5g total fat
(0.5g saturated fat); 782kJ
(187 cal); 33.9g carbohydrate;
7.4g protein; 2.9g fibre
tip Try using our cranberry and almond granola recipe (page 31) instead of the toasted muesli for a breakfast sensation.

You need about four trimmed rhubarb stalks for this recipe.

2 cups (220g) coarsely chopped
   fresh or frozen rhubarb
¼ cup (55g) caster sugar
½ cup (125ml) water
½ teaspoon ground cinnamon
1⅓ cups (375g) low-fat
   vanilla yogurt
⅓ cup (50g) toasted muesli

1 Combine rhubarb, sugar, the water and cinnamon in medium saucepan; bring to a boil. Reduce heat; simmer, uncovered, stirring occasionally, about 10 minutes or until rhubarb is tender. Transfer to medium heatproof bowl, cover; refrigerate 1 hour.
2 Divide rhubarb mixture among four ¾-cup (180ml) serving glasses; top with yogurt then muesli.

did you know? Calcium is well absorbed from dairy products, but poorly absorbed from foods rich in oxalic acid, such as spinach and rhubarb. So stick to dairy foods as the main source of dietary calcium, but enjoy rhubarb as a tangy, vibrant, stewed fruit.

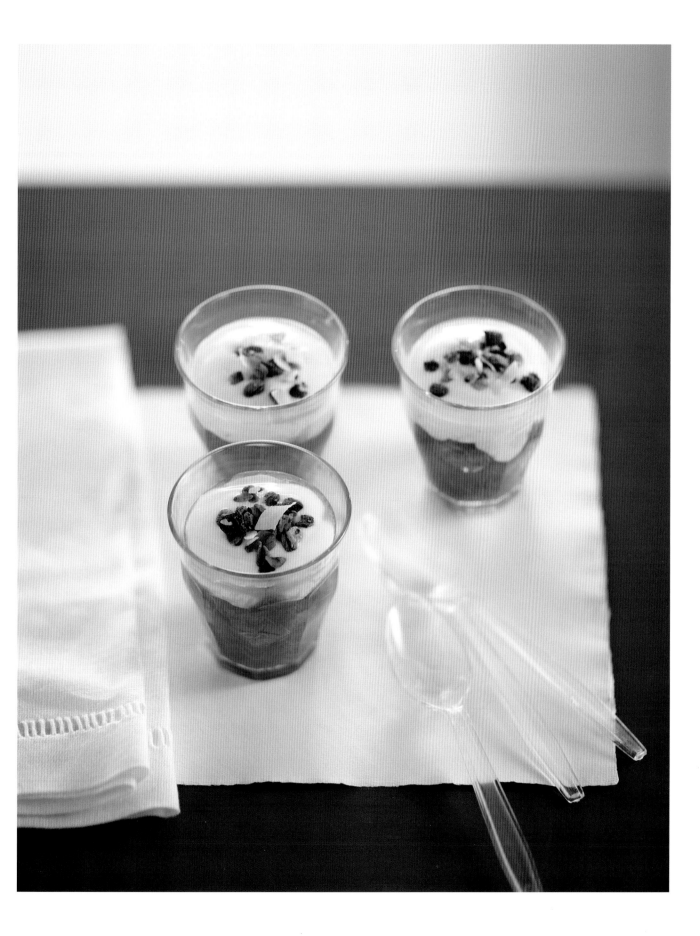

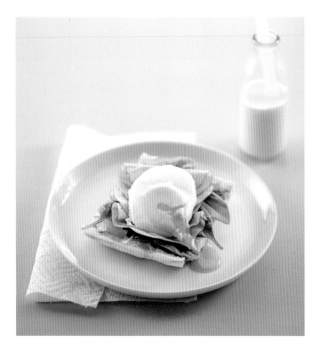

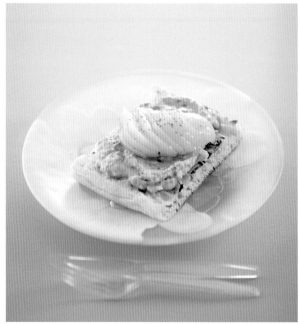

spinach, ham and poached egg

preparation time 5 minutes cooking time 5 minutes serves 4
per serving 8.4g total fat (2.4g saturated fat); 1062kJ
(254 cal); 24.3g carbohydrate; 18.9g protein; 1.9g fibre

4 eggs
½ large loaf turkish bread (215g), halved
75g baby spinach leaves
150g shaved ham

1 Half-fill large frying pan with water; bring to a boil.
Break one egg into a cup then slide into pan; repeat
with remaining eggs. When all eggs are in pan, allow
water to return to a boil. Cover pan, turn off heat; stand
about 4 minutes or until a light film of egg white sets over
yolks. Remove eggs, one at a time, using slotted spoon;
place spoon on absorbent-paper-lined saucer to blot up
poaching liquid.
2 Meanwhile, cut bread pieces horizontally; toast cut
sides. Top toast with spinach, ham and eggs.

honeyed ricotta and pears

preparation time 5 minutes cooking time 5 minutes serves 4
per serving 7g total fat (3.6g saturated fat); 1397kJ
(330 cal); 52.7g carbohydrate; 11.8g protein; 3.9g fibre

1 cup (240g) reduced-fat ricotta cheese
2 tablespoons honey
¼ teaspoon finely grated orange rind
¼ teaspoon ground cinnamon
½ large loaf turkish bread (215g), halved
825g can sliced pears, drained, sliced
1 tablespoon honey, extra

1 Preheat grill.
2 Combine ricotta, honey, rind and cinnamon in
small bowl.
3 Meanwhile, cut bread pieces horizontally; toast cut
sides. Spread ricotta mixture onto toast, top with pear;
grill about 2 minutes or until hot. Drizzle with extra honey.

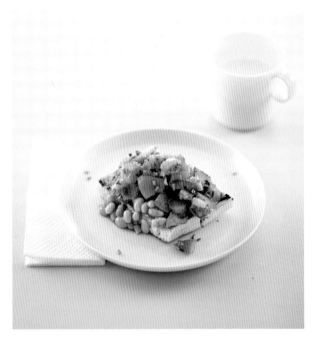

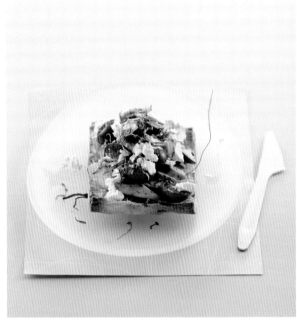

baked beans, bacon, tomato and chives

preparation time 5 minutes cooking time 5 minutes serves 4
per serving 10.4g total fat (3.2g saturated fat); 1450kJ
(347 cal); 34.5g carbohydrate; 22g protein; 7.4g fibre

2 medium tomatoes (300g), chopped coarsely
1 tablespoon finely chopped chives
420g can baked beans in tomato sauce
4 rindless bacon rashers (240g), chopped coarsely
½ large loaf turkish bread (215g), halved

1 Preheat grill.
2 Combine tomato and chives in small bowl.
3 Heat beans in small saucepan.
4 Meanwhile, cook bacon, stirring, in heated small frying pan until crisp; drain on absorbent paper.
5 Cut bread pieces horizontally; toast cut sides. Top toast with beans, bacon and tomato mixture; grill about 2 minutes or until hot.

roasted cherry tomatoes, fetta, avocado and basil

preparation time 5 minutes cooking time 10 minutes serves 4
per serving 15.4g total fat (4.7g saturated fat); 1237kJ
(296 cal); 25.6g carbohydrate; 12.4g protein; 3.1g fibre

250g cherry tomatoes, halved
½ large loaf turkish bread (215g), halved
1 medium avocado (250g), sliced thinly
100g piece reduced-fat fetta cheese, crumbled
¼ cup coarsely chopped fresh basil

1 Preheat grill.
2 Grill tomato about 5 minutes or until softened.
3 Meanwhile, cut bread pieces horizontally; toast cut sides. Top toast with avocado, tomato and cheese; grill about 2 minutes or until hot. Serve sprinkled with basil.

porridge with honeyed coconut and dried fruit

preparation time 10 minutes
cooking time 15 minutes **serves** 4
per serving 6.2g total fat
(4g saturated fat); 1233kJ
(295 cal); 47.7g carbohydrate;
7.3g protein; 4.1g fibre

This bowl of homely goodness is made even better with the addition of dried fruits and coconut.
Porridge has a low GI rating, meaning it will keep young tummies full for hours.

½ cup (25g) flaked coconut
¼ cup (90g) honey
1⅓ cups (330ml) low-fat milk
1 cup (250ml) water
1 cup (90g) rolled oats
¼ cup (35g) finely chopped
  dried pears
2 tablespoons finely
  chopped sultanas
2 tablespoons finely chopped
  dried apricots

1 Preheat oven to 180°C/160°C fan-forced. Line shallow medium baking dish with baking paper.
2 Sprinkle coconut into dish; drizzle with 1 tablespoon of the honey. Cook, uncovered, about 5 minutes or until browned lightly. Cool in dish.
3 Meanwhile, stir milk, the water and oats in medium saucepan over medium heat about 10 minutes or until porridge is thick and creamy. Stir in remaining honey and half the dried fruit.
4 Serve porridge, sprinkled with remaining fruit and coconut, with warmed milk, if you like.

did you know? Rolled oats in muesli and porridge contain a special type of soluble fibre known as beta-glucan that has powerful cholesterol-lowering properties. So start your kids on the oats habit as early as possible, and set them up for a heart-healthy life.

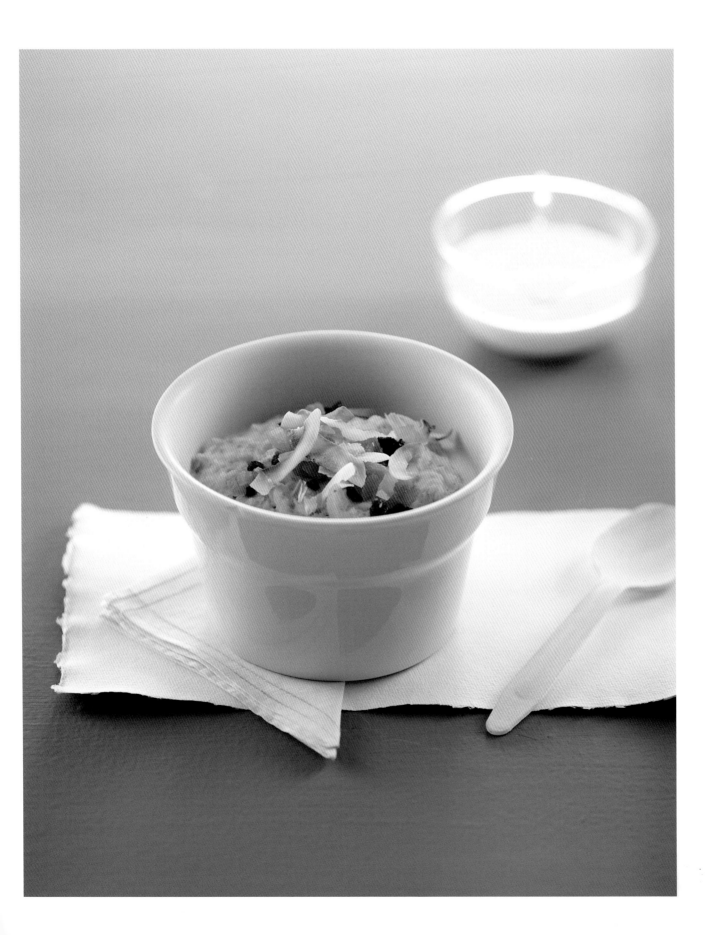

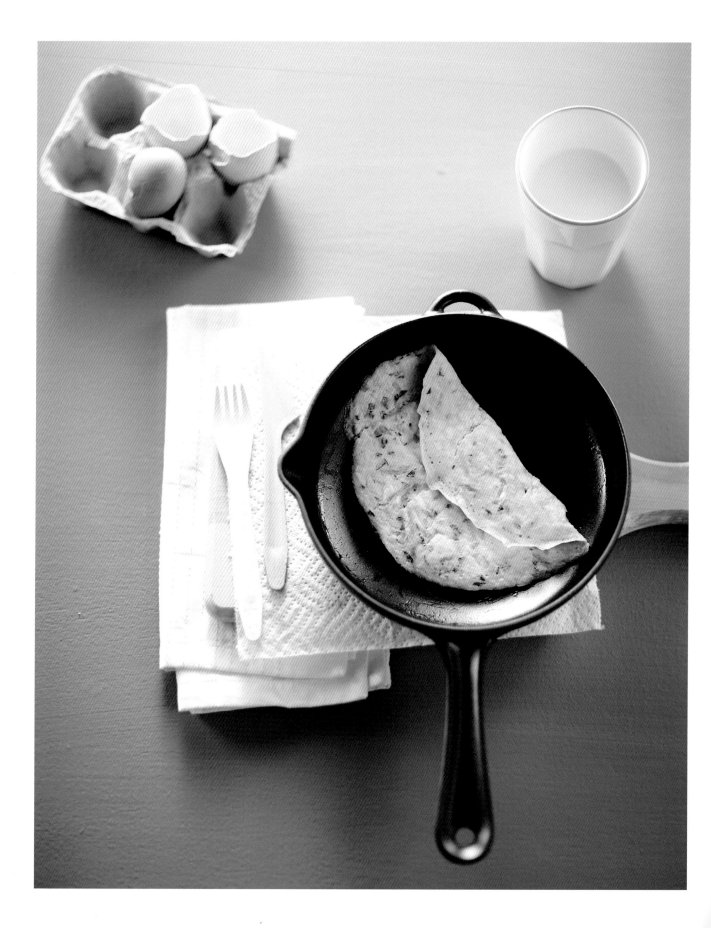

corn, cheese and carrot omelettes

preparation time 10 minutes
cooking time 20 minutes **serves** 4
per serving 14.7g total fat
(5.6g saturated fat); 1162kJ
(278 cal); 15.3g carbohydrate;
19.6g protein; 4g fibre

*A quick and easy before-school
tummy-filler. Add a bit of crisp
bacon or even a few pan-fried
mushrooms to the omelette,
if you like.*

8 eggs
310g can creamed corn
1 large carrot (180g),
    grated coarsely
¼ cup finely chopped fresh
    flat-leaf parsley
½ cup (60g) coarsely grated
    reduced-fat cheddar cheese

1 Whisk eggs in medium bowl until combined; stir in remaining ingredients.
2 Pour a quarter of the egg mixture into heated oiled small frying pan; cook over medium heat until omelette is set. Fold omelette in half, slide onto plate; cover to keep warm.
3 Repeat process with remaining egg mixture to make four omelettes.

did you know? New research is confirming that the naturally occurring cholesterol in eggs doesn't raise blood cholesterol to the extent of the "bad" type of fats known as saturated and trans fats. That's why the Heart Foundation now has awarded eggs with a tick of approval, and for most people (especially kids) an egg a day is okay.

juices & smoothies

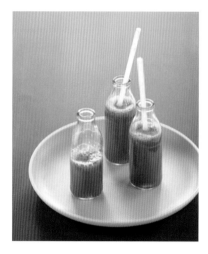

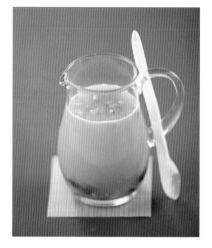

melonade

preparation time 10 minutes
(plus standing time)
makes 1 litre (4 cups)
per 1 cup (250ml) 0.3g total fat
(0.8g saturated fat); 301kJ
(72 cal); 16.1g carbohydrate;
0.6g protein; 0.8g fibre

*You need a 1kg piece of watermelon
for this recipe.*

½ cup (125ml) lemon juice
2 tablespoons caster sugar
3 cups (500g) coarsely
    chopped watermelon
1½ cups (375ml) chilled sparkling
    mineral water

1 Combine juice and sugar in
small saucepan; stir over low heat
until sugar dissolves. Cool.
2 Blend or process watermelon,
in batches, until smooth; strain
through sieve into large jug. Stir
in lemon syrup and mineral water;
serve immediately.

passionfruit sparkler

preparation time 10 minutes
(plus freezing time) **makes** 1 litre (4 cups)
per 1 cup (250ml) 0.5g total fat
(0g saturated fat); 723kJ
(173 cal); 31.1g carbohydrate;
4.1g protein; 13.2g fibre

2 x 170g cans passionfruit in syrup
1 medium orange (240g), segmented
150g seedless red grapes, halved
1½ cups (375ml) pineapple juice
1½ cups (375ml) orange juice
1 cup (250ml) sparkling mineral water

1 Freeze passionfruit in syrup in
ice-cube trays.
2 Combine passionfruit cubes with
remaining ingredients in large jug.

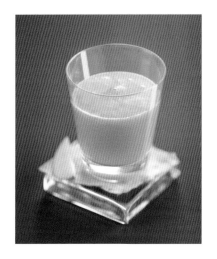 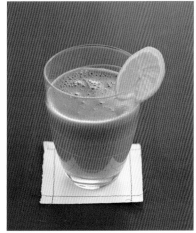 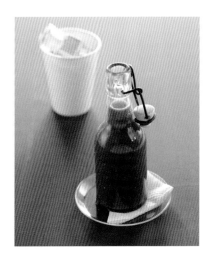

apple, pear and ginger juice

preparation time 5 minutes
makes 1 cup (250ml)
per serving 0.3g total fat
(0g saturated fat); 823kJ
(197 cal); 43.1g carbohydrate;
1g protein; 0.2g fibre

*We used a green-skinned apple here,
but any variety is suitable for this drink.*

1 medium unpeeled apple (150g),
   cored, cut into wedges
1 medium unpeeled pear (230g),
   cored, cut into wedges
1cm piece fresh ginger (5g)

1 Push apple, pear and ginger
through juice extractor into glass.
2 Serve with ice.

carrot, orange and ginger juice

preparation time 5 minutes
makes 1 cup (250ml)
per serving 0.3g total fat
(0g saturated fat); 506kJ
(121 cal); 22.6g carbohydrate;
3g protein; 0.2g fibre

1 large orange (300g),
   peeled, quartered
1 medium carrot (120g),
   chopped coarsely
1cm piece fresh ginger (5g)

1 Push orange carrot and ginger
through juice extractor into glass.
2 Serve with ice.

peach and raspberry juice

preparation time 5 minutes
makes 1 cup (250ml)
per serving 0.3g total fat
(0.6g saturated fat); 314kJ
(75 cal); 13.7g carbohydrate;
1.9g protein; 4.1g fibre

1 large peach (220g), peeled
   chopped coarsely
¼ cup (35g) fresh or
   frozen raspberries
½ cup (125ml) water

1 Blend or process peach and
raspberries until smooth; pour
into glass.
2 Stir in the water; serve with ice.

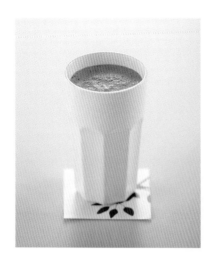

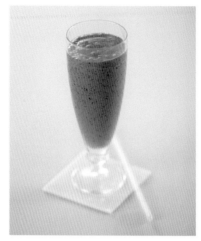

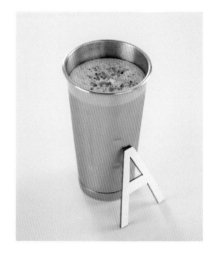

strawberry soy smoothie

preparation time 5 minutes
makes 1 cup (250ml)
per serving 5.6g total fat
(0.6g saturated fat); 744kJ
(178 cal); 24.7g carbohydrate;
5g protein; 4.2g fibre

5 strawberries (100g), hulled, halved
½ cup (125ml) chilled strawberry
  soy milk
½ cup (125ml) strawberry
  soy ice-cream

1 Blend or process ingredients
until smooth.
2 Pour into glass; serve immediately.

brekky berry smoothie

preparation time 5 minutes
makes 1 cup (250ml)
per serving 0.8g total fat
(0.2g saturated fat); 765kJ
(183 cal); 28.7g carbohydrate;
13.1g protein; 3.3g fibre

½ cup (75g) frozen mixed berries
½ cup (125ml) chilled
  low-fat milk
¼ cup (70g) low-fat vanilla yogurt
1 Weet-Bix (15g)

1 Blend or process ingredients
until smooth.
2 Pour into glass; serve immediately.

choc-malt smoothie

preparation time 5 minutes
makes 1¼ cups (310ml)
per serving 12.4g total fat
(6.8g saturated fat); 1254kJ
(360 cal); 47.8g carbohydrate;
13.9g protein; 0.1g fibre

½ cup (125ml) chilled
low-fat milk
1 cup (250ml) reduced-fat
  vanilla ice-cream
1 tablespoon malted milk powder
2 teaspoons chocolate-
  hazelnut spread
pinch ground cinnamon

1 Blend or process ingredients
until smooth.
2 Pour into glass; serve immediately.

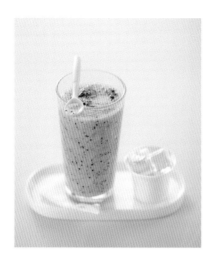

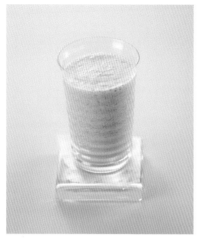

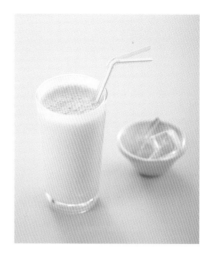

kiwifruit and mint frappé

preparation time 5 minutes
makes 1½ cups (375ml)
per serving 0.8g total fat
(0g saturated fat); 974kJ
(233 cal); 44.8g carbohydrate;
5.2g protein; 12.2g fibre

4 medium kiwifruits (340g), peeled, chopped coarsely
¾ cup ice cubes
¼ cup (60ml) apple juice
¼ cup coarsely chopped fresh mint leaves
1 teaspoon caster sugar
1 teaspoon finely shredded fresh mint

1 Blend or process kiwifruit, ice, juice, chopped mint and sugar until smooth.
2 Pour into glass; top with shredded mint.

almond and berry smoothie

preparation time 5 minutes
makes 1 cup (250ml)
per serving 7g total fat
(4.5g saturated fat); 1630kJ
(370 cal); 59g carbohydrate;
15.5g protein; 2.7g fibre

1 cup (250ml) chilled water
½ cup (70g) roasted slivered almonds
3 drops vanilla extract
⅓ cup (50g) frozen raspberries
¾ cup (180ml) reduced-fat frozen raspberry yogurt

1 Blend or process the water and nuts until smooth. Strain mixture into small jug; discard solids.
2 Return almond milk to blender with vanilla, raspberries and yogurt; blend until smooth.
3 Pour into glass; serve immediately.

buttermilk fruit smoothie

preparation time 5 minutes
makes 1 cup (250ml)
per serving 2.8g total fat
(1.7g saturated fat); 1488kJ
(356 cal); 71.2g carbohydrate;
7.5g protein; 6g fibre

Freeze unpeeled bananas then use them straight from the freezer to give your smoothie an ice-creamy texture.

1 small pear (180g), cored, chopped coarsely
1 small banana (130g), chopped coarsely
2 teaspoons honey
½ cup (125ml) chilled buttermilk
½ cup (125ml) chilled apple juice

1 Blend or process ingredients until smooth.
2 Pour into glass; serve with ice.

lunchboxes

Each of these recipes makes 4 and can be prepared in less than half an hour.

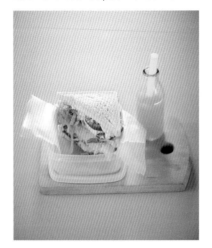 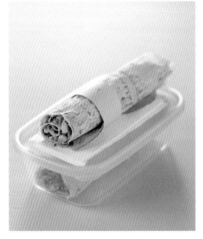 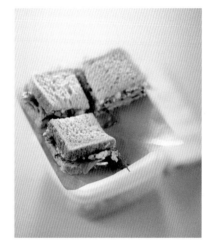

egg salad sandwich

per sandwich 13.6g total fat
(4g saturated fat); 1622kJ
(388 cal); 44.8g carbohydrate;
19.5g protein; 3.7g fibre
tip Filling can be refrigerated
for up to two days.

Combine 6 finely chopped hard-boiled
eggs, 1 finely chopped celery stalk,
1 finely sliced green onion, 2 tablespoons
finely grated parmesan cheese and
¼ cup low-fat mayonnaise in medium
bowl. Sandwich egg mixture, 1 cup
shredded iceberg lettuce and 2 sliced
egg tomatoes between 8 slices of
white bread.

guacamole and ham wrap

per wrap 23.2g total fat
(5.2g saturated fat); 1877kJ
(449 cal); 40.1g carbohydrate;
17.9g protein; 4.7g fibre

Mash 2 avocados with 1 tablespoon
lime juice in small bowl. Stir in
1 small finely chopped seeded
tomato, 1 tablespoon finely chopped
fresh chives and a drained 130g can
corn kernels. Spread 4 pieces lavash
bread with guacamole; sprinkle with
200g shaved ham then roll tightly
to enclose filling.

cheese and salad sandwich

per sandwich 6g total fat
(2.3g saturated fat); 911kJ
(218 cal); 20.9g carbohydrate;
17.5g protein; 4.5g fibre

Combine 200g low-fat cottage
cheese, ⅓ cup coarsely grated
reduced-fat cheddar cheese, 1 cup
shredded baby spinach leaves, 1 thinly
sliced green onion, 1 finely grated
small carrot, 1 tablespoon roasted
sesame seeds and 2 teaspoons
lemon juice in medium bowl.
Sandwich 30g mesclun and
cheese mixture between 8 slices
of wholemeal bread.

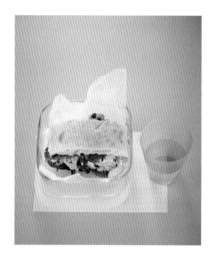

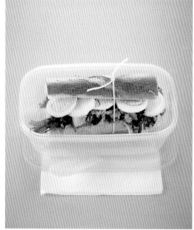

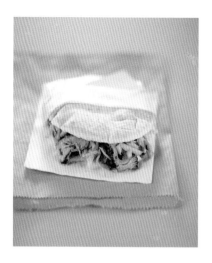

apricot chicken on turkish

per sandwich 23g total fat
(4g saturated fat); 2533kJ
(606 cal); 61.2g carbohydrate;
35.5g protein; 5.3g fibre
tip Filling can be refrigerated
for up to two days.

Combine 2 chicken breast fillets,
2 teaspoons moroccan spice mix
and 1 tablespoon olive oil in medium
bowl. Peel and slice a small kumara.
Cook chicken and kumara in heated
oiled medium frying pan until cooked;
cool. Slice chicken; combine with
⅓ cup low-fat yogurt and 2 tablespoons
each low-fat mayonnaise, finely
chopped dried apricots and slivered
almonds in medium bowl. Quarter
large loaf of turkish bread; split
quarters in half. Sandwich 30g baby
rocket leaves, kumara and chicken
mixture between bread pieces.

mediterranean tuna baguette

per baguette 15.7g total fat
(2.9g saturated fat); 1781kJ
(426 cal); 47.9g carbohydrate;
20.9g protein; 4.2g fibre
tip Filling can be refrigerated
for up to two days.

Cook 1 diced medium potato until
tender; drain. Shake 2 tablespoons
olive oil, 1 tablespoon red wine
vinegar and 1 teaspoon dijon
mustard together in screw-top jar.
Combine potato and dressing with
1 tablespoon finely chopped black
olives, 1 finely chopped seeded
medium tomato and a drained 185g
can tuna in springwater in medium
bowl. Halve 2 small french sticks
crossways then split in half.
Sandwich 30g mesclun, 2 sliced
hard-boiled eggs and tuna mixture
between bread pieces.

roast beef and slaw pockets

per pocket 17.2g total fat
(4.2g saturated fat); 1923kJ
(460 cal); 48.1g carbohydrate;
25.3g protein; 5.3g fibre
tip Filling can be refrigerated
for up to two days.

Shake 2 tablespoons olive oil,
2 teaspoons dijon mustard and
2 tablespoons each white wine
vinegar and water together in
screw-top jar. Combine dressing
with 2 cups finely shredded cabbage,
1 finely chopped small red onion,
1 finely grated small carrot and ¼ cup
coarsely chopped fresh flat-leaf
parsley in medium bowl. Split
4 pocket pitta breads a little more
than halfway through; fill pockets
with slaw and 200g sliced roast beef.

Each of these recipes serves one and can be prepared in under 25 minutes.

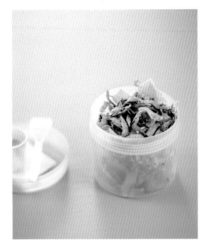

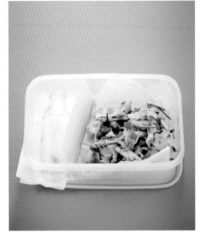

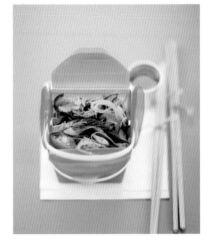

pork and cabbage salad

per serving 21.2g total fat (3.6g saturated fat); 1436kJ (342 cal); 8.8g carbohydrate; 26.2g protein; 6.9g fibre

You need ⅛ small wombok and ⅛ small red cabbage. Use leftover roast pork or chinese barbecued pork.

Shake 1 tablespoon olive oil, 2 teaspoons apple cider vinegar and ½ teaspoon dijon mustard together in screw-top jar. Using vegetable peeler, slice 1 small carrot into ribbons; combine in medium bowl with ¾ cup each of finely shredded wombok and finely shredded red cabbage, 1 thinly sliced green onion and ½ cup shredded leftover pork. Pack salad and dressing in separate containers in lunchbox.

chicken pasta salad

per serving 16.9g total fat (7.4g saturated fat); 5008kJ (1198 cal); 198g carbohydrate; 53.9g protein; 13.1g fibre

Boil ¾ cup farfalle pasta in water until tender; drain. Melt 10g butter in small frying pan; cook 1 crushed garlic clove, 50g thinly sliced mushrooms and 1 small finely chopped medium red capsicum until tender. Shake 2 teaspoons red wine vinegar and 1 teaspoon wholegrain mustard together in screw-top jar. Combine pasta and vegetable mixture in medium bowl with ½ cup shredded barbecued chicken and 1 tablespoon finely chopped fresh chives. Pack salad and dressing in separate containers in lunchbox.

thai beef noodle salad

per serving 22.8g total fat (7.9g saturated fat); 1768kJ (423 cal); 16.2g carbohydrate; 36.8g protein; 3.1g fibre

Cook 150g beef rump steak in heated oiled small frying pan. Cover, stand 10 minutes then slice thinly. Place 20g bean thread noodles in medium heatproof bowl, cover with boiling water; stand until tender, drain, cut into random lengths. Combine sliced beef and noodles in same bowl with ¼ sliced seeded lebanese cucumber, 25g halved cherry tomatoes, ¼ thinly sliced small red capsicum and 1 thinly sliced green onion. Shake ¼ cup fresh mint leaves, 2 teaspoons each peanut oil, sweet chilli sauce and lime juice together in screw-top jar. Pack salad and dressing in separate containers in lunchbox.

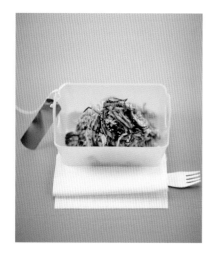

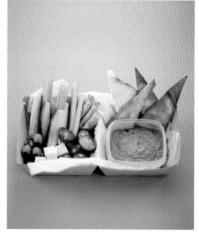

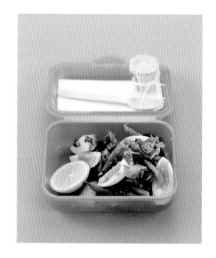

teriyaki chicken rice salad

per serving 7.7g total fat
(1.8g saturated fat); 1538kJ
(368 cal); 47.8g carbohydrate;
23.7g protein; 5g fibre

Rinse ¼ cup koshihikari rice in cold water until water is almost clear; drain. Place rice and ¼ cup water in small saucepan, cover; bring to a boil. Reduce heat; simmer, covered, about 10 minutes. Remove from heat; stand rice, covered, until cool. Combine rice with 1 tablespoon rice vinegar, 2 teaspoons teriyaki sauce and 1cm piece grated fresh ginger in medium bowl. Add ½ cup shredded barbecued chicken, half a coarsely chopped seeded lebanese cucumber, 1 coarsely grated small carrot and 1 teaspoon roasted sesame seeds; mix well. Pack in container sprinkled with ¼ sheet shredded toasted seaweed and another teaspoon of roasted sesame seeds.

beetroot dip and antipasto

per serving 18.7g total fat
(9.8g saturated fat); 2324kJ
(556 cal); 59.4g carbohydrate;
30.4g protein; 10.2g fibre

Preheat oven to 180°C/160°C fan-forced. Cut 1 large pitta bread into thin triangles; toast on oven tray about 8 minutes or until crisp. Meanwhile, blend or process a drained 225g can beetroot slices and 1 tablespoon low-fat sour cream until smooth. Separately pack half the dip and half the lavash crisps (keep the remaining halves of each for another lunch) with 1 tablespoon drained green stuffed olives, 100g halved cherry tomatoes, 50g shaved ham, 40g cubed low-fat cheddar cheese, half a thinly sliced celery stalk and ¼ thinly sliced lebanese cucumber.

niçoise salad

per serving 7.8g total fat
(2.4g saturated fat); 1179kJ
(282 cal); 20.3g carbohydrate;
29.7g protein; 4.9g fibre

Cook 100g quartered baby new potatoes and 50g halved green beans, separately, until tender. Rinse under cold water; drain. Combine potato and beans with a 95g can drained and flaked tuna in springwater, 1 quartered hard-boiled egg, 1 tablespoon each seeded black olives and coarsely chopped fresh flat-leaf parsley in medium bowl. Pack salad with half a lemon.

snacks

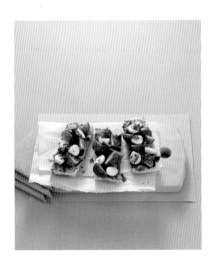

bruschetta fingers

preparation time 5 minutes
cooking time 5 minutes **serves** 1
per serving 12.2g total fat
(4.4g saturated fat); 1618kJ
(387 cal); 50.6g carbohydrate;
16.3g protein; 4.3g fibre

1 small turkish bread roll (110g)
2 teaspoons sun-dried
  tomato pesto
6 cherry tomatoes (60g),
  quartered
30g baby bocconcini cheese,
  sliced thinly
1 tablespoon finely chopped
  fresh flat-leaf parsley

1 Split bread in half; toast, cut-side
up, then cut into fingers.
2 Spread toasted sides of bread
with pesto; top with tomato and
cheese then sprinkle with parsley.

did you know? Snacks should make up at least a third of your child's food intake, so pack healthy, portable snacks in the lunchbox, with extras on sport days.

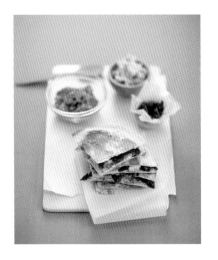

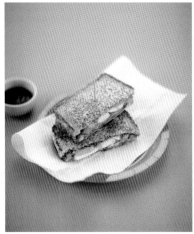

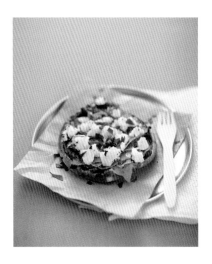

chicken quesadilla

preparation time 5 minutes
cooking time 5 minutes **serves** 1
per serving 41.2g total fat
(11.6g saturated fat); 3265kJ
(781 cal); 61.8g carbohydrate;
36.5g protein; 9.1g fibre

2 large flour tortillas
40g packaged reduced-fat
  cream cheese
½ cup (80g) shredded
  barbecued chicken
¼ cup (35g) coarsely chopped
  drained semi-dried tomatoes
½ medium avocado (125g), mashed

1 Place one tortilla on board;
spread with cream cheese then
top with chicken and tomato.
2 Spread second tortilla with
avocado; place, avocado-side-
down, on first tortilla.
3 Toast in sandwich press until
golden brown. Serve quesadilla
cut into quarters.

ham, egg and cheese toastie

preparation time 5 minutes
cooking time 5 minutes **serves** 1
per serving 16.1g total fat
(6.9g saturated fat); 1898kJ
(454 cal); 44.3g carbohydrate;
29.7g protein; 5.9g fibre

2 slices wholemeal bread (90g)
1 tablespoon barbecue sauce
30g shaved ham
1 hard-boiled egg, sliced
¼ cup (30g) coarsely grated
  reduced-fat cheddar cheese

1 Spread bread with sauce; top
one bread slice with ham, egg and
cheese then remaining bread slice.
2 Toast in sandwich press until
golden brown.

pumpkin and fetta pizza

preparation time 10 minutes
cooking time 15 minutes **serves** 1
per serving 10.7g total fat
(3.4g saturated fat); 1576kJ
(377 cal); 51.6g carbohydrate;
16.1g protein; 3.9g fibre

50g piece pumpkin
1 teaspoon olive oil
1 pocket pitta bread (85g)
2 tablespoons bottled tomato
  pasta sauce
25g reduced-fat fetta
  cheese, crumbled
2 teaspoons finely chopped
  fresh mint

1 Preheat oven to 180°C/160°C
fan-forced.
2 Using vegetable peeler, slice
pumpkin into thin strips. Combine
pumpkin and oil in small bowl.
3 Spread pitta with sauce; top
with pumpkin and cheese. Cook
about 15 minutes or until pumpkin
is tender. Serve sprinkled with mint.

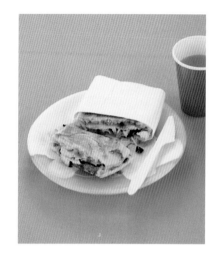

turkey on toasted turkish

preparation time 5 minutes
cooking time 5 minutes **serves** 1
per serving 7g total fat
(2.2g saturated fat); 1659kJ
(397 cal); 58.5g carbohydrate;
22.4g protein; 3.1g fibre

1 tablespoon cranberry sauce
1 small turkish bread roll (110g)
30g shaved turkey
10g shaved reduced-fat
   jarlsberg cheese
10g baby spinach leaves

1 Split bread in half. Spread sauce
onto cut sides then sandwich turkey,
cheese and spinach between pieces.
2 Toast in sandwich press until
golden brown.

did you know? Even though Popeye claimed to boost his energy levels with spinach, this might not be that accurate. Iron is needed for the formation of red blood cells and to carry oxygen around the body, but the form of plant iron in spinach is not that easy to absorb. Spinach is, however, still a nutritious vegetable so, parents, keep this fact to yourself.

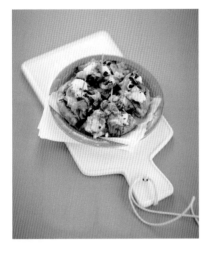
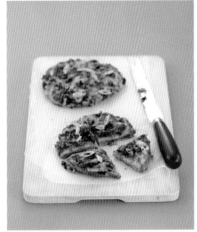
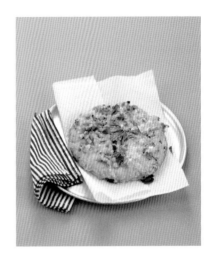

pesto, ham and mushroom pizza

preparation time 5 minutes
cooking time 15 minutes **serves** 1
per serving 15.6g total fat
(5.4g saturated fat); 1848kJ
(442 cal); 45.4g carbohydrate;
27.9g protein; 3.8g fibre

3 large button mushrooms (30g),
   chopped finely
1 tablespoon basil pesto
1 pocket pitta bread (85g)
25g ham, chopped finely
1 tablespoon pizza cheese
2 tablespoons low-fat
   cottage cheese
1 tablespoon finely chopped
   fresh flat-leaf parsley

1 Preheat oven to 180°C/160°C
fan-forced.
2 Combine mushrooms and pesto
in small bowl. Spread pitta with
mushroom mixture; top with ham and
cheeses. Cook about 15 minutes or
until cheese melts. Sprinkle parsley
over pizza just before serving.

pizza mexicana

preparation time 5 minutes
cooking time 15 minutes **serves** 1
per serving 9.5g total fat
(4.7g saturated fat); 1689kJ
(404 cal); 54.7g carbohydrate;
21g protein; 6.6g fibre

1 pocket pitta bread (85g)
¼ cup (60g) canned refried beans
¼ small red capsicum (35g),
   chopped finely
2 teaspoons sweet chilli sauce
2 tablespoons pizza cheese
1 green onion, sliced thinly

1 Preheat oven to 180°C/160°C
fan-forced.
2 Spread pitta with beans; top with
capsicum, sauce and cheese. Cook
about 15 minutes or until cheese
melts. Sprinkle onion over pizza just
before serving.

bacon and corn pizza

preparation time 5 minutes
cooking time 15 minutes **serves** 1
per serving 17.3g total fat
(7.7g saturated fat); 2027kJ
(485 cal); 50.5g carbohydrate;
29.7g protein; 3g fibre

1 pocket pitta bread (85g)
1 tablespoon corn relish
1 rasher rindless bacon (65g),
   chopped finely
2 tablespoons pizza cheese
1 tablespoon finely chopped
   fresh flat-leaf parsley

1 Preheat oven to 180°C/160°C
fan-forced.
2 Spread pitta with relish; top with
bacon and cheese. Cook about
15 minutes or until bacon crisps and
cheese melts. Sprinkle parsley over
pizza just before serving.

mains

veal schnitzel, potato smash and roasted tomatoes

preparation time 15 minutes
cooking time 15 minutes **serves** 4
per serving 10.1g total fat
(3.7g saturated fat); 1956kJ
(468 cal); 57.5g carbohydrate;
32.6g protein; 7g fibre

*Potato smash is a great way to do
something different with potatoes; it's
easy to prepare and yummy to eat.*

1kg baby new potatoes, unpeeled
20g butter
1 tablespoon low-fat milk
1 cup (70g) stale breadcrumbs
⅓ cup (55g) cornflake crumbs
2 tablespoons finely chopped
   fresh oregano
2 teaspoons finely grated
   lemon rind
4 x 100g veal schnitzels
1 egg white, beaten lightly
cooking-oil spray
250g baby vine-ripened
   truss tomatoes

1 Preheat oven to 200°C/180°C
fan-forced. Oil two oven trays.
2 Boil, steam or microwave
potatoes until tender; drain. Mash
about half the potatoes in medium
bowl with butter and milk until smooth.
Add remaining potatoes to bowl;
crush roughly with fork. Cover to
keep warm.
3 Combine crumbs, oregano and
rind in medium bowl. Coat schnitzels,
one at a time, in egg white then crumb
mixture. Spray with cooking-oil;
place on trays with tomatoes. Cook,
about 10 minutes or until schnitzels
are cooked through. Serve schnitzels
and tomatoes with smash.

did you know? Cooking tomatoes with a little oil, especially olive oil, boosts lycopene absorption. Lycopene is a potent antioxidant that protects body cells from damage by free radicals.

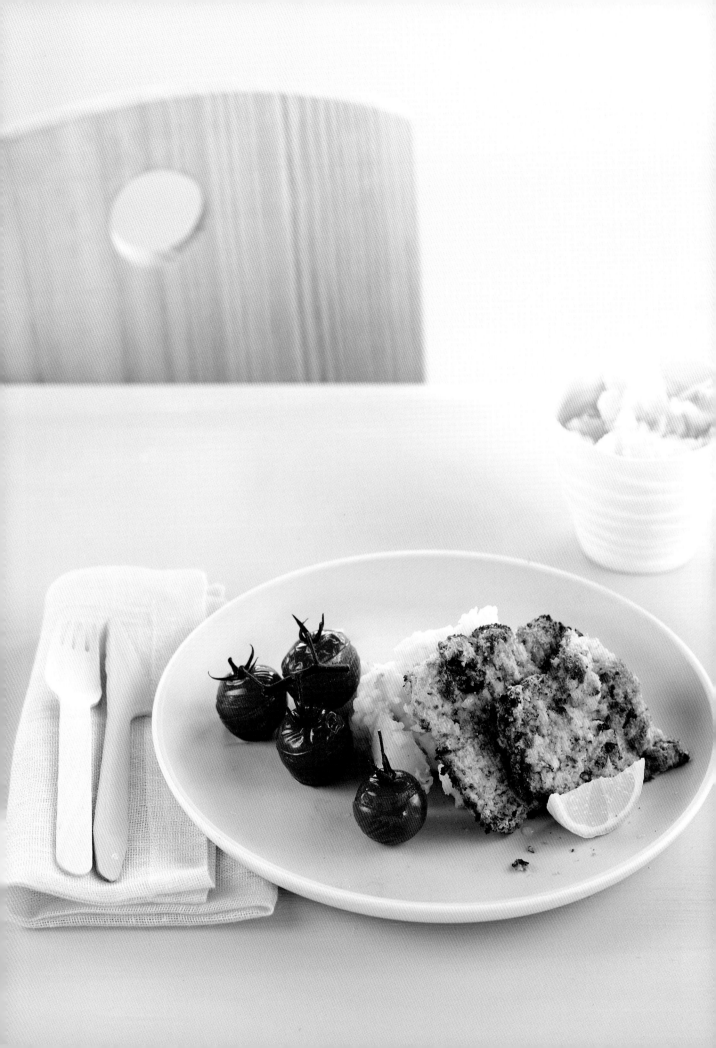

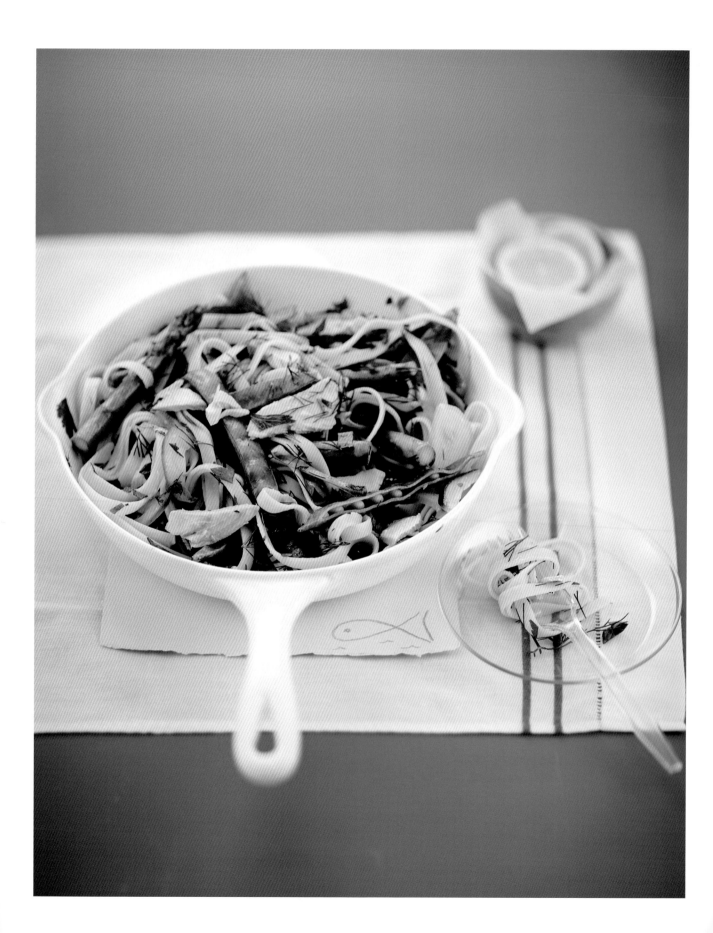

pasta primavera with poached salmon

preparation time 25 minutes
cooking time 15 minutes **serves** 4
per serving 13.2g total fat
(4.7g saturated fat); 2324kJ
(556 cal); 69.8g carbohydrate;
35.5g protein; 6.3g fibre

375g fettuccine
1.25 litres (5 cups) water
440g salmon fillets
2 sprigs fresh dill
6 black peppercorns
2 teaspoons finely grated
    lemon rind
20g butter
2 cloves garlic, crushed
1 medium red onion (170g),
    sliced thinly
170g asparagus, halved crossways
½ cup (60g) frozen peas
150g snow peas, trimmed, halved
2 tablespoons lemon juice
2 teaspoons finely chopped
    fresh dill
2 tablespoons coarsely chopped
    fresh flat-leaf parsley

1 Cook pasta in large saucepan of boiling water, uncovered, until just tender; drain.

2 Meanwhile, combine the water, fish, dill, peppercorns and half the rind in large saucepan; bring to a boil. Reduce heat; simmer, uncovered, 8 minutes, turning fish halfway through cooking time. Remove fish from poaching liquid. When cool enough to handle, discard skin; flake fish in medium bowl.

3 Heat butter in same cleaned pan; cook garlic, onion and asparagus until asparagus is just tender. Add peas, pasta, remaining rind, fish and juice; stir until hot. Toss in herbs just before serving.

did you know? Salmon is richer than tuna in essential omega-3 fatty acids. When going for omega-3s you can also boost intakes with fortified foods, just look on the label for the terms DHA or EPA, which describe the best form of omegas.

beef enchiladas

preparation time 45 minutes
cooking time 30 minutes **serves** 4
per serving 26.7g total fat
(9.2g saturated fat); 2696kJ
(645 cal); 57.4g carbohydrate;
38.8g protein; 10.1g fibre

2 tablespoons olive oil
1 small yellow capsicum (150g),
  chopped finely
1 small red onion (100g),
  chopped finely
1 clove garlic, crushed
1 teaspoon ground cumin
½ teaspoon sweet paprika
400g beef mince
2 tablespoons tomato paste
2 tablespoons water
130g can kidney beans,
  rinsed, drained
2 tablespoons coarsely chopped
  fresh oregano
2 cups (500ml) bottled tomato
  pasta sauce
1 cup (250ml) water, extra
10 x 15cm corn tortillas
1 cup (120g) coarsely grated
  reduced-fat cheddar cheese
1 tablespoon finely chopped
  fresh flat-leaf parsley

1 Heat half the oil in large frying pan; cook capsicum, half the onion and half the garlic, stirring, until vegetables soften. Add spices; cook, stirring, until fragrant. Add mince; cook, stirring, until changed in colour. Stir in paste and the 2 tablespoons water; simmer, stirring, 1 minute. Place filling mixture in large heatproof bowl; stir in beans and oregano.

2 Heat remaining oil in same pan; cook remaining onion and garlic, stirring, until onion softens. Add pasta sauce and the extra water; bring to a boil. Reduce heat; simmer, uncovered, 5 minutes.

3 Preheat oven to 180°C/160°C fan-forced. Oil shallow square 3-litre (12-cup) ovenproof dish. Spread ½ cup pasta sauce mixture in dish.

4 Warm tortillas according to package instructions. Dip tortillas, one at a time, in pasta sauce mixture; place on board. Divide filling among tortillas, placing mixture on edge of tortilla; roll tortillas to enclose filling.

5 Place enchiladas, seam-side down, snugly in single layer, in dish. Spread remaining pasta sauce mixture over enchiladas; sprinkle with cheese. Cook, uncovered, about 15 minutes or until enchiladas are hot.

6 Serve enchiladas sprinkled with parsley and, if you like, separate small bowls of sour cream, shredded lettuce and chopped tomatoes.

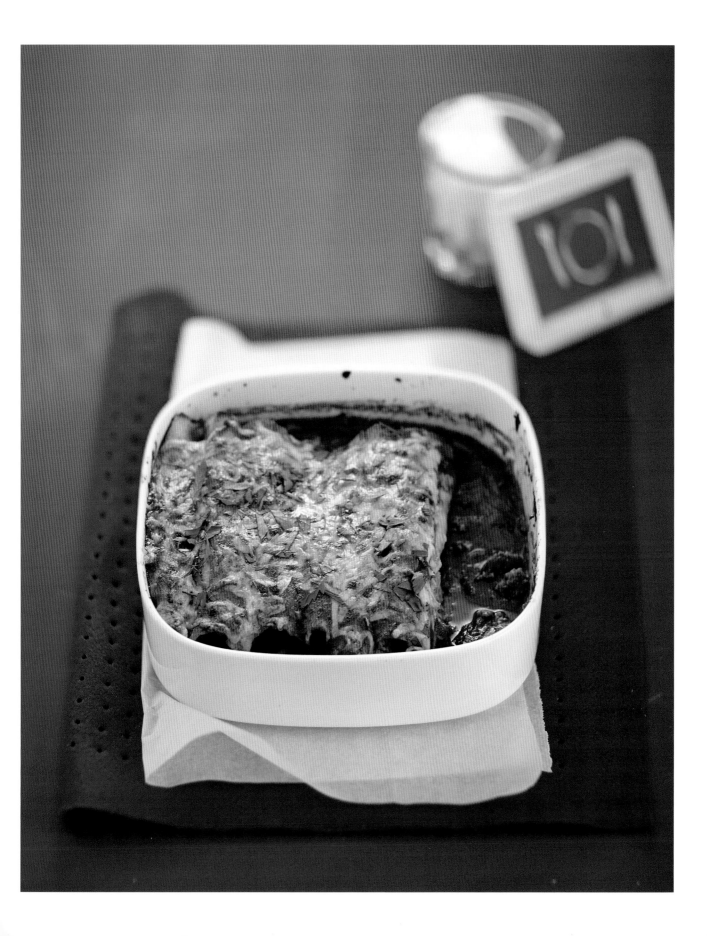

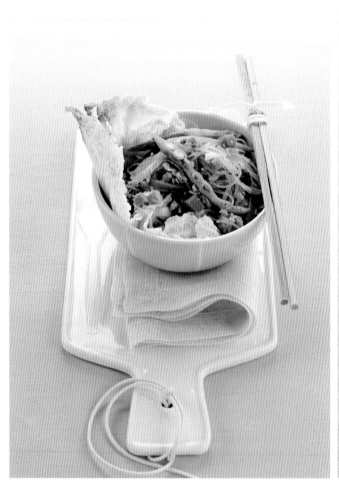

chicken sang choy bow

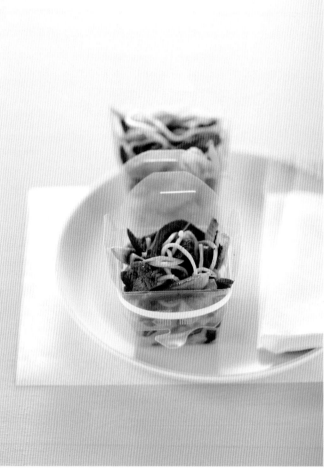

hokkien chilli beef

chicken sang choy bow

preparation time 10 minutes
cooking time 10 minutes serves 4
per serving 13.7g total fat
(3.4g saturated fat); 1572kJ
(376 cal); 29.9g carbohydrate;
29.7g protein; 6.3g fibre

Remove eight large outer leaves from trimmed wombok, before shredding.

100g rice stick noodles
2 teaspoons vegetable oil
500g chicken mince
1 medium red onion (170g),
    chopped finely
1 tablespoon curry powder
1 large carrot (180g), chopped finely
2 tablespoons oyster sauce
2 tablespoons char siu sauce
½ small wombok (350g),
    shredded coarsely
100g snow peas, sliced lengthways
8 large wombok leaves

1 Place noodles in medium heatproof bowl, cover with boiling water; stand 3 minutes, drain. Cut into random lengths.
2 Heat oil in wok; stir-fry mince and onion until mince changes colour. Add curry powder; stir-fry until fragrant. Add carrot; stir-fry until carrot softens.
3 Add sauces, wombok and peas to wok; stir-fry about 2 minutes or until vegetables soften.
4 Divide wombok leaves among serving bowls. Toss noodles with mince mixture; divide among wombok cups.

hokkien chilli beef

preparation time 15 minutes
(plus refrigeration time)
cooking time 15 minutes serves 4
per serving 17g total fat
(5.7g saturated); 2771kJ
(663 cal); 75.7g carbohydrate;
47.9g protein; 5.9g fibre

¼ cup (60ml) sweet chilli sauce
2 tablespoons plum sauce
600g piece beef rump steak,
    sliced thinly
450g hokkien noodles
1 tablespoon peanut oil
4 green onions, cut into 2cm lengths
1 clove garlic, crushed
1 medium red capsicum (200g),
    sliced thinly
115g baby corn, halved lengthways
150g sugar snap peas, trimmed
½ cup (125ml) vegetable stock

1 Combine sauces with beef in medium bowl, cover; refrigerate 3 hours.
2 Meanwhile, place noodles in medium heatproof bowl, cover with boiling water; separate with fork, drain.
3 Heat oil in wok; stir-fry beef mixture, in batches, until browned.
4 Stir-fry onion and garlic in wok until onion browns. Add capsicum and corn; stir-fry until vegetables are almost softened. Return beef to wok with noodles, peas and stock; stir-fry until hot.

coconut-fish and chips with lemon coriander mayo

preparation time 25 minutes
cooking time 40 minutes **serves** 4
per serving 12.9g total fat
(5.1g saturated); 2186kJ
(523 cal); 55.6g carbohydrate;
41.6g protein; 7.2g fibre

Fish is a terrific source of nutrition for growing bodies, and our lower-in-fat version of fish and chips is so tasty everyone will be fighting for the last piece. We've used perch, but you can use any firm white fish you like.

1kg coliban potatoes
cooking-oil spray
⅓ cup (25g) desiccated coconut
¾ cup (50g) stale
    breadcrumbs, toasted
2 teaspoons finely grated
    lemon rind
2 egg whites
1 tablespoon low-fat milk
4 perch fillets (720g)
¼ cup (35g) plain flour
lemon coriander mayo
½ cup (150g) low-fat mayonnaise
1 tablespoon finely chopped
    fresh coriander
2 teaspoons finely
    grated lemon rind
1 tablespoon lemon juice

1 Preheat oven to 220°C/200°C fan-forced.
2 Cut potatoes into 1cm-thick slices; cut slices into 1cm-thick chips. Place chips, in single layer, on baking-paper-lined oven tray; spray with cooking oil. Roast about 40 minutes or until browned and crisp.
3 Meanwhile, combine coconut, breadcrumbs and rind in shallow medium bowl. Whisk egg whites and milk in another shallow medium bowl. Coat fish in flour; shake off excess. Dip fish in egg white mixture then coat in breadcrumb mixture. Place on baking-paper-lined oven tray; spray with cooking-oil. Cook for final 20 minutes of chips' cooking time.
4 Combine ingredients for lemon coriander mayo in small bowl. Serve mayo with fish and chips.

did you know? A weekly intake of 2-3 fish meals is recommended to ensure that essential omega-3 fats are sufficient in the diet. The average intake for 12-18 year olds is around 200mg of omega-3 per day, which is less than half recommended levels.

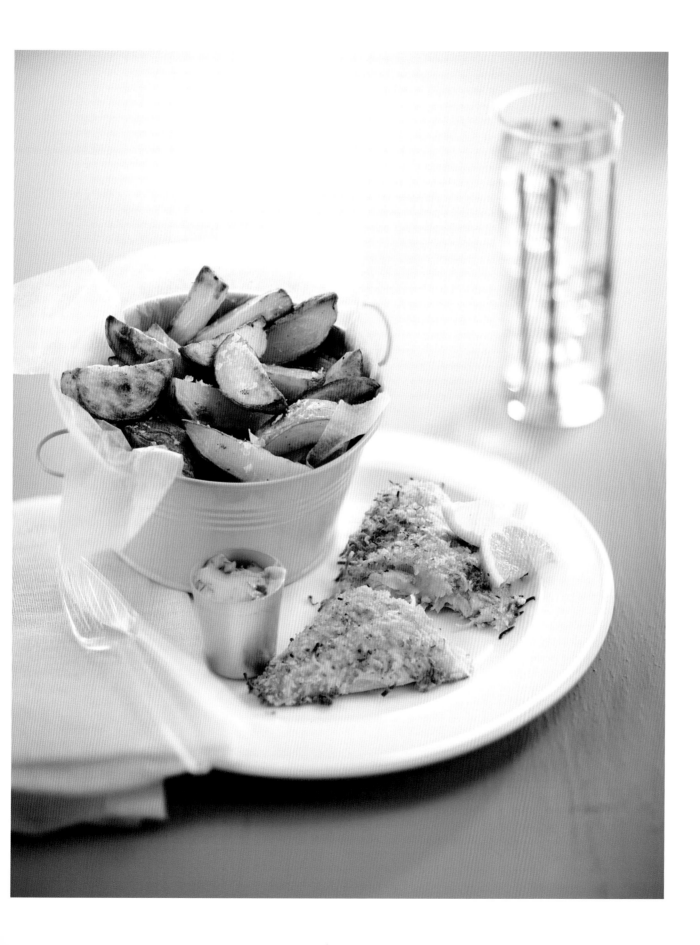

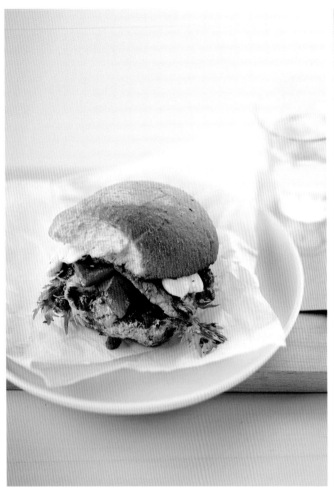

grilled steak and vegie-salsa sandwich

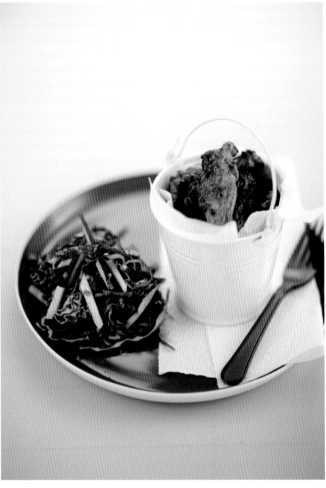

finger lickin' chicken wings with pink coleslaw

grilled steak and vegie-salsa sandwich

preparation time 5 minutes
cooking time 25 minutes **serves** 4
per serving 18.8g total fat
(6.6g saturated fat); 2245kJ
(537 cal); 52.8g carbohydrate;
36.2g protein; 5.1g fibre

1 medium red capsicum (200g),
    chopped coarsely
1 small zucchini (90g),
    chopped coarsely
1 medium red onion (170g),
    chopped coarsely
2 tablespoons prepared
    chunky tomato salsa
4 beef minute steaks (400g)
4 wholemeal hamburger buns (360g)
1 tablespoon olive oil
40g mesclun
120g bocconcini cheese,
    sliced thickly

1 Cook capsicum, zucchini and onion on heated oiled grill plate until tender; combine with salsa in small bowl.
2 Cook steak on heated oiled grill plate until cooked as desired.
3 Preheat grill.
4 Meanwhile, halve buns horizontally; brush cut-sides with oil. Toast bun halves, cut-sides up, under grill.
5 Place mesclun and vegie-salsa on bottom halves of buns; top with steaks then cheese. Grill about 2 minutes or until cheese melts. Top with remaining bun halves.

finger lickin' chicken wings with pink coleslaw

preparation time 20 minutes
(plus cooling and refrigeration time)
cooking time 50 minutes **serves** 6
per serving 14.9g total fat
(3.6g saturated fat); 1785kJ
(427 cal); 31.9g carbohydrate;
38.6g protein; 4.3g fibre

1 cup (250ml) tomato sauce
¼ cup (60ml) worcestershire sauce
⅓ cup (75g) firmly packed
    brown sugar
¼ cup (60ml) apple cider vinegar
2 tablespoons american mustard
2 cloves garlic, crushed
12 large chicken wings (1.5kg)
pink coleslaw
1 large red apple (200g)
¼ medium red cabbage (350g),
    shredded finely
½ cup coarsely chopped fresh mint
2 tablespoons olive oil
1 tablespoon red wine vinegar
1 teaspoon dijon mustard

1 Combine sauces, sugar, vinegar, mustard and garlic in medium saucepan; bring to a boil. Remove marinade from heat; cool marinade to room temperature.
2 Cut wings into three pieces at joints; discard tips. Combine chicken with marinade in large bowl, cover; refrigerate 3 hours or overnight.
3 Preheat oven to 220°C/200°C fan-forced.
4 Place chicken, in single layer, in large shallow baking dish; brush marinade over chicken. Cook, uncovered, turning occasionally, about 45 minutes or until chicken is browned and cooked through.
5 Meanwhile, make pink coleslaw. Serve coleslaw with chicken wings.
pink coleslaw Core unpeeled apple; cut into matchsticks. Place apple in large bowl with remaining ingredients; toss to combine.

chicken vegetable soup with croutons

preparation time 20 minutes
cooking time 25 minutes **serves** 6
per serving 11.4g total fat
(4g saturated fat); 1434kJ
(343 cal); 27.7g carbohydrate;
29.7g protein; 5.6g fibre

You can use any shaped cutter you like for the croutons, or simply cut the bread into cubes.

1 tablespoon olive oil
1 medium brown onion (150g), chopped finely
1 clove garlic, crushed
2 medium tomatoes (300g), chopped finely
400g chicken breast fillets, sliced thinly
450g piece pumpkin, cut into fine dice
2 litres (8 cups) chicken stock
2 slices wholemeal bread (90g)
420g can borlotti beans, rinsed, drained
150g broccoli, cut into florets
½ cup (40g) coarsely grated parmesan cheese

1 Preheat oven to 180°C/160°C fan-forced.
2 Heat half the oil in large saucepan; cook onion, garlic and tomato, stirring, until onion softens. Add chicken, pumpkin and stock; bring to a boil. Reduce heat; simmer, uncovered, about 10 minutes or until pumpkin is almost tender.
3 Meanwhile, cut bread into shapes with cutter; combine bread and remaining oil in small bowl. Place bread, in single layer, on oven tray; toast, in oven, until croutons are crisp.
4 Add beans and broccoli to soup; cook, uncovered, about 3 minutes or until heated through.
5 Serve soup topped with croutons and sprinkled with cheese.

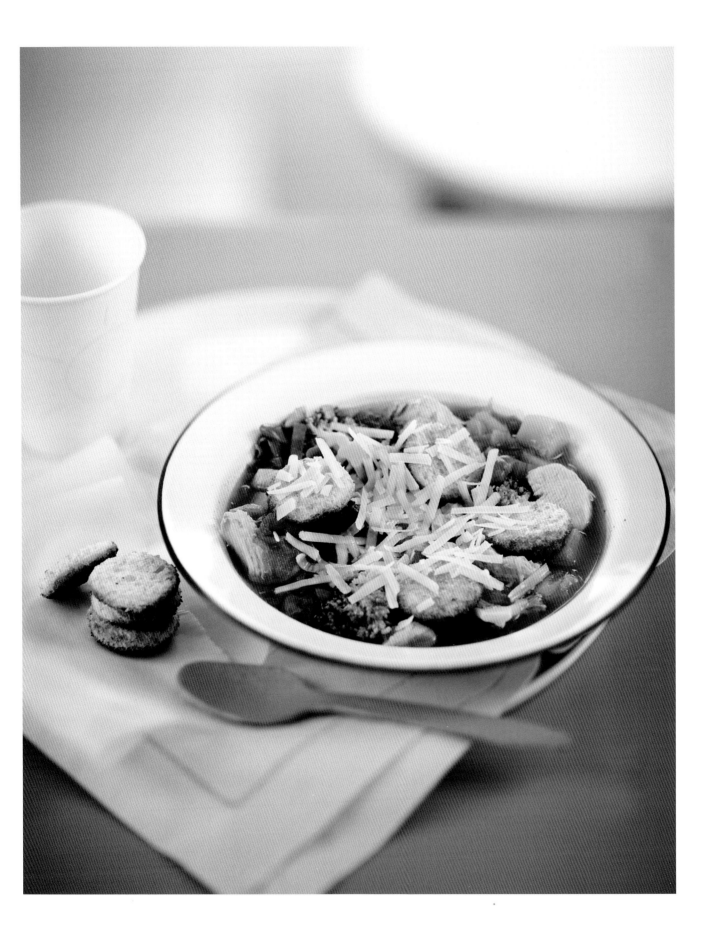

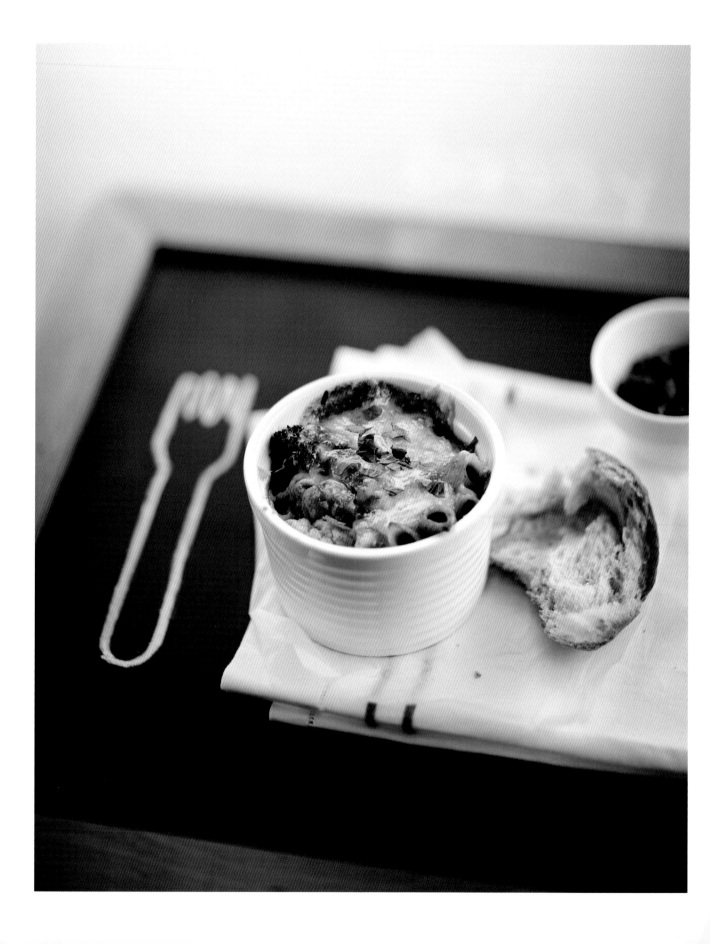

cheesy-vegie pasta bake

preparation time 15 minutes
cooking time 20 minutes **serves** 6
per serving 10.9g total fat
(5.4g saturated fat); 1952kJ
(467 cal); 62.3g carbohydrate;
25.5g protein; 7.4g fibre

375g penne
300g broccoli, cut into florets
500g cauliflower, cut into florets
2 teaspoons vegetable oil
1 large brown onion (200g),
    chopped finely
1 teaspoon mustard powder
1 teaspoon sweet paprika
¼ cup (35g) plain flour
1½ cups (375ml) low-fat milk
420g can tomato soup
400g can diced tomatoes
1½ cups (180g) coarsely grated
    reduced-fat cheddar cheese
2 tablespoons finely chopped
    fresh flat-leaf parsley

1 Cook pasta in large saucepan of boiling water, uncovered, until just tender; drain. Cover to keep warm.
2 Meanwhile, cook broccoli and cauliflower in medium saucepan of boiling water, uncovered, until tender; drain. Cover to keep warm.
3 Preheat grill.
4 Heat oil in same large pan; cook onion, stirring, until softened. Add mustard, paprika and flour; cook, stirring, over low heat, 2 minutes. Gradually stir in milk and soup; stir over heat until mixture boils and thickens. Add undrained tomatoes; cook, stirring, until mixture is hot.
5 Stir pasta, broccoli, cauliflower and 1 cup of the cheese into tomato mixture. Divide pasta mixture among six 1-cup (250ml) flameproof dishes, sprinkle with remaining cheese; grill until cheese melts and is browned lightly. Sprinkle pasta bake with parsley just before serving.

did you know? Cauliflower and broccoli belong to the Brassica family and contain potent anti-cancer compounds known as the glucosinolates. Other family members include brussels sprouts and cabbage.

minestrone with meatballs

preparation time 30 minutes
cooking time 45 minutes **serves** 6
per serving 14.6g total fat
(3.9g saturated fat); 1572kJ
(376 cal); 33.4g carbohydrate;
26.2g protein; 5.6g fibre

Everybody loves meatballs so your kids won't complain about having to eat their vegetables when they see these yummy meatballs in their bowls.
Many varieties of cooked white beans are available canned, among them cannellini, butter and haricot, any of which is suitable for this recipe.

1 tablespoon olive oil
1 large brown onion (200g), chopped finely
2 cloves garlic, crushed
1 large carrot (180g), diced into 1cm pieces
2 trimmed celery stalks (200g), diced into 1cm pieces
2 tablespoons tomato paste
2 cups (500ml) chicken stock
400g can crushed tomatoes
1½ cups (375ml) water
425g can white beans, rinsed, drained
½ cup (180g) small pasta shells
2 tablespoons finely chopped fresh oregano
meatballs
500g beef mince
1 small brown onion (80g), chopped finely
2 cloves garlic, crushed
½ cup (35g) stale breadcrumbs
1 egg
1 tablespoon olive oil

1 Make meatballs.
2 Heat oil in large saucepan; cook onion and garlic, stirring, until onion softens. Add carrot and celery; cook, stirring, about 5 minutes or until vegetables are tender. Add paste; cook, stirring, 2 minutes.
3 Add stock, undrained tomatoes and the water; bring to a boil. Add meatballs, beans and pasta, reduce heat; simmer, uncovered, about 20 minutes or until meatballs are cooked through. Serve soup sprinkled with oregano.
meatballs Combine mince, onion, garlic, breadcrumbs and egg in medium bowl; roll level tablespoons of mixture into balls. Heat oil in large frying pan; cook meatballs, in batches, until browned.

did you know? Herbs and spices are starting to capture greater attention by the scientific community. New research shows that herbs and spices can boost your daily antioxidant levels, with cinnamon, clove, oregano, peppermint and thyme in the top five for antioxidant activity.

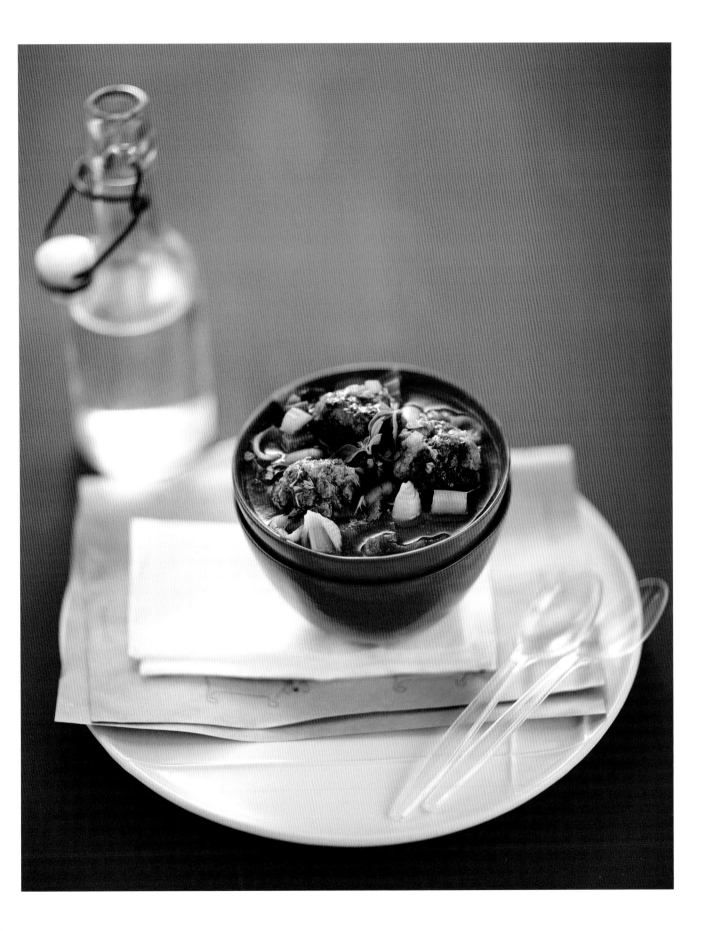

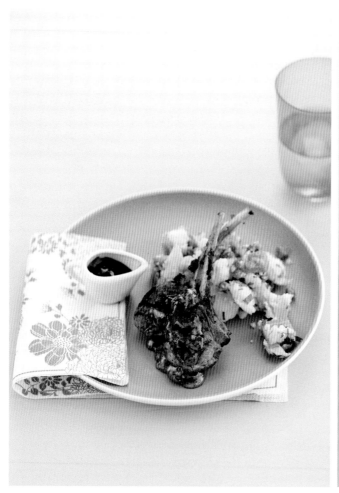

minty lamb cutlets with mixed vegie smash

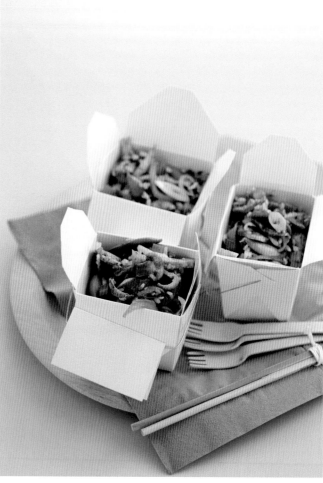

pork fried rice

minty lamb cutlets with mixed vegie smash

preparation time 10 minutes
cooking time 30 minutes **serves** 4
per serving 15.8g total fat
(4.9g saturated fat); 1572kJ
(376 cal); 38.4g carbohydrate;
16.3g protein; 7.3g fibre

1 tablespoon finely chopped
   fresh mint
⅓ cup (110g) mint jelly
1 teaspoon finely grated lemon rind
2 teaspoons olive oil
8 french-trimmed lamb cutlets (400g)
mixed vegie smash
600g baby new potatoes, halved
2 large carrots (360g), diced into
   2cm pieces
1 cup (120g) frozen peas
1 tablespoon olive oil
1 tablespoon lemon juice
2 tablespoons finely chopped
   fresh mint

1 Make mixed vegie smash.
2 Combine mint and jelly in
small bowl.
3 Rub combined rind and oil over
lamb; cook lamb on heated oiled
grill plate (or grill or barbecue) until
cooked as desired.
4 Serve lamb with smash and
mint mixture.
mixed vegie smash Boil, steam or
microwave potato, carrot and peas,
separately, until tender; drain. Crush
potato and peas roughly in large bowl;
stir in carrot and remaining ingredients.

pork fried rice

preparation time 15 minutes
cooking time 20 minutes **serves** 4
per serving 13g total fat
(3.7g saturated fat); 1726kJ
(413 cal); 42.8g carbohydrate;
28.2g protein; 5.2g fibre

*We've used brown long-grain rice in this
recipe because of its lovely nutty taste,
but you can replace it with white long-
grain rice if you wish. You need to cook
about 1⅓ cups rice for this recipe.*

3 teaspoons peanut oil
2 eggs, beaten lightly
1 medium brown onion (150g),
   sliced thinly
1 clove garlic, crushed
2 rashers rindless bacon (130g),
   sliced thinly
200g pork fillet, sliced thinly
150g mushrooms, quartered
150g sugar snap peas, trimmed,
   halved crossways
1 medium carrot (120g),
   chopped finely
3 cups cold cooked brown
   long-grain rice
2 tablespoons kecap manis
4 green onions, sliced thinly

1 Heat one teaspoon of the oil in
wok. Pour half the egg into wok;
cook over medium heat, tilting wok,
until almost set. Remove omelette
from wok; roll tightly, slice thinly.
Repeat using another teaspoon of
oil and remaining egg.
2 Heat remaining oil in wok; stir-fry
onion and garlic until onion softens.
Add bacon and pork; stir-fry until
bacon is crisp. Add mushrooms, peas
and carrot; stir-fry about 3 minutes
or until carrot is just tender.
3 Add rice and kecap to wok; stir-fry
until hot. Toss omelette and onion
through fried rice just before serving.

rosemary-scented lamb shanks with almond couscous

preparation time 5 minutes
cooking time 6 hours 15 minutes
serves 4
per serving 14.4g total fat
(4.4g saturated fat); 2972kJ
(711 cal); 66.1g carbohydrate;
75.5g protein; 4.9g fibre

2 large brown onions (400g),
   unpeeled, chopped coarsely
9 cloves garlic, unpeeled,
   chopped coarsely
1½ cups (375ml) chicken stock
1½ cups (375ml) water
6 stalks fresh rosemary
8 french-trimmed lamb shanks (2kg)
10g butter
2 teaspoons plain flour
almond couscous
¾ cup (180ml) water
¾ cup (180ml) chicken stock
1½ cups (300g) couscous
⅓ cup (45g) roasted
   slivered almonds
1 cup coarsely chopped fresh
   flat-leaf parsley

1 Preheat oven to 160°C/140°C fan-forced.
2 Combine onion, garlic, stock and the water in large deep baking dish; top with rosemary then lamb. Cover tightly with foil; cook 6 hours, turning lamb after 3 hours. Remove lamb from baking dish; cover to keep warm.
3 Meanwhile, make almond couscous.
4 Using back of spoon, work butter into flour in small bowl. Strain juice from baking dish into small saucepan; discard solids. Skim fat from juice; discard fat. Bring juice to a boil. Reduce heat; whisk in flour mixture until sauce boils and thickens slightly.
5 Serve lamb with couscous and sauce.
almond couscous Bring the water and stock to a boil in medium saucepan. Remove from heat; stir in couscous. Cover; stand about 5 minutes or until liquid is absorbed, fluffing with fork occasionally. Stir in nuts and parsley.

did you know? Food neophobia is the term used to describe a fear of new foods. (Neophobia is the fear of new things or experiences.) It's very common in children, especially toddlers, and research shows that you may have to present a new food or taste, like chilli, up to nine times before a child will accept it.

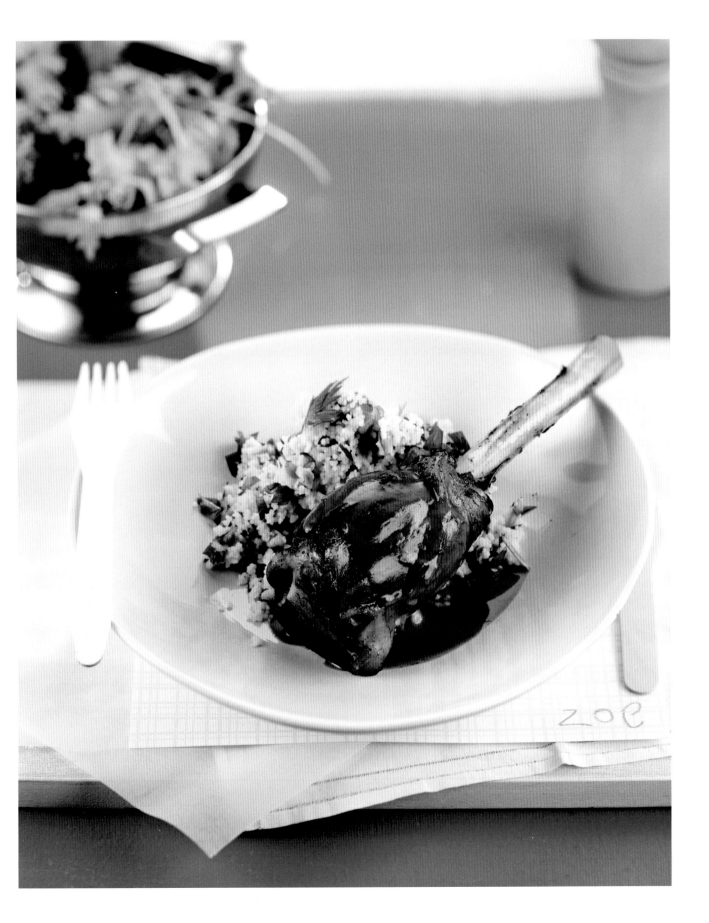

Each of these recipes serves 4 and can be on the table in under 40 minutes.

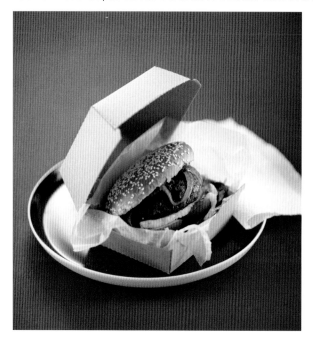

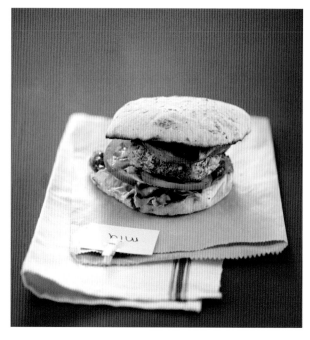

beef burgers

per serving 12.3g total fat (4.1g saturated fat); 2337kJ
(559 cal); 71.8g carbohydrate; 35.7g protein; 6.9g fibre

1 small red onion (100g), halved
500g beef mince
½ cup (125ml) barbecue sauce
1 tablespoon tomato sauce
4 thin slices fresh pineapple (150g)
4 hamburger buns (360g)
1½ cups finely shredded iceberg lettuce
1 large tomato (220g), sliced thinly
225g can beetroot slices, drained

1 Chop half of the onion finely; cut remaining half into
four slices.
2 Combine mince, 1 tablespoon of the barbecue sauce,
tomato sauce and chopped onion in medium bowl. Shape
mixture into four patties.
3 Cook pineapple slices and onion slices on heated oiled
grill plate until pineapple is browned. Cook patties.
4 Split buns; toast, cut-sides up, under preheated grill.
5 Spread remaining barbecue sauce on bun bases; layer
all ingredients between bun halves.

italian chicken patties on foccaccia

per serving 18.6g total fat (5.5g saturated fat); 2667kJ
(638 cal); 72.4g carbohydrate; 41g protein; 6.6g fibre

500g chicken mince
⅓ cup (50g) drained semi-dried tomatoes, chopped finely
½ small brown onion (40g), chopped finely
¼ cup (20g) coarsely grated parmesan cheese
2 tablespoons finely chopped fresh flat-leaf parsley
4 slices pancetta (60g)
4 foccaccia rolls (440g)
½ cup (160g) tomato chutney
40g mixed baby salad leaves
1 large tomato (220g), sliced thinly

1 Combine mince, semi-dried tomato, onion, cheese and
parsley in medium bowl. Shape mixture into four patties.
2 Cook pancetta in heated large frying pan until crisp;
remove from pan. Cook patties in same pan.
3 Split rolls; toast, cut-sides up, under preheated grill.
4 Spread chutney on roll bases; sandwich leaves, tomato,
patties and pancetta between roll halves.

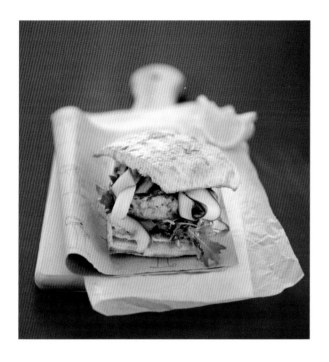

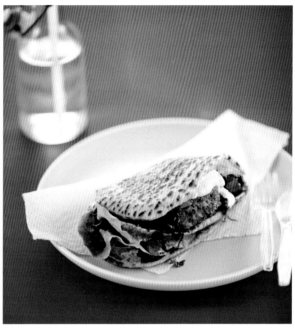

lemon salmon patties on turkish bread

per serving 10.6g total fat (2.5g saturated fat); 2203kJ (527 cal); 70.3g carbohydrate; 33.5g protein; 6.2g fibre

500g pontiac potatoes, chopped coarsely
415g can pink salmon, drained
1 egg
2 green onions, chopped finely
1 teaspoon finely grated lemon rind
1 lebanese cucumber (130g)
1 large loaf turkish bread (430g), cut into quarters
⅓ cup (80ml) sweet chilli sauce
40g mizuna

1 Cook potato until tender; drain; mash potato.
2 Combine salmon, egg, onion and rind in medium bowl with potato. Shape mixture into four patties.
3 Cook patties in heated oiled large frying pan.
4 Using a vegetable peeler, slice cucumber into ribbons.
5 Split bread; toast, cut-sides up, under preheated grill.
6 Spread sauce on bread bases; sandwich cucumber, mizuna and patties between bread.

pitta filled with lamb and tabbouleh

per serving 15.7g total fat (5.2g saturated fat); 2132kJ (510 cal); 49.9g carbohydrate; 39.3g protein; 4.7g fibre

¾ cup (200g) low-fat yogurt
2 cloves garlic, crushed
500g lamb mince
1 teaspoon ground cumin
1 teaspoon ground coriander
½ small brown onion (40g), chopped finely
1 egg
4 pitta pockets (340g)
½ baby cos lettuce (90g), leaves separated
⅔ cup (115g) tabbouleh

1 Combine yogurt and half the garlic in small bowl.
2 Combine remaining garlic, mince, spices, onion and egg in medium bowl. Shape into eight patties.
3 Cook patties in heated oiled large frying pan.
4 Split pitta not quite through; fill pockets with lettuce, tabbouleh, patties and yogurt.

sides

Each of these recipes serves 4 and can be on the table in 40 minutes.

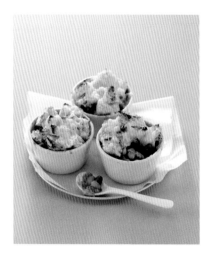

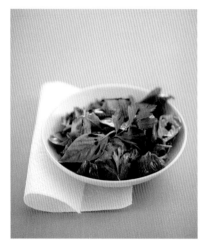

tomato and bean bake

per serving 12.5g total fat (5.2g saturated fat); 1195kJ (286 cal); 22.4g carbohydrate; 17g protein; 8g fibre

Heat 2 teaspoons olive oil in medium saucepan; cook 1 chopped small brown onion and 100g chopped trimmed green beans. Add a 420g can rinsed and drained four-bean mix, 250g halved cherry tomatoes, 2 tablespoons tomato paste and ½ cup water; cook until tomato softens. Preheat grill. Combine 2 teaspoons olive oil, 90g chopped wholemeal bread and ½ cup pizza cheese in small bowl. Stir 2 tablespoons chopped fresh basil into bean mixture; spoon mixture into four 1-cup (250ml) shallow flameproof dishes, top with bread mixture. Grill until bread is brown and crisp.

tomato and capsicum salad

per serving 9.7g total fat (1.3g saturated fat); 640kJ (153 cal); 9.7g carbohydrate; 4.7g protein; 4.8g fibre

Preheat grill. Chop 2 large red capsicums; combine in medium bowl with 1 tablespoon olive oil and 1 crushed garlic clove. Grill capsicum about 10 minutes or until tender. Cut 5 medium tomatoes into six wedges each; combine in same bowl with 1 tablespoon olive oil and 1 crushed garlic clove. Grill tomato about 5 minutes or until tender. Combine ⅓ cup each firmly packed fresh basil and fresh flat-leaf parsley, 40g baby spinach leaves, 2 teaspoons balsamic vinegar, tomato and capsicum in large bowl.

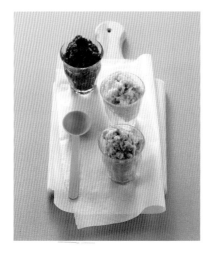

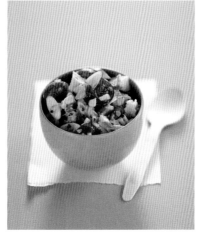

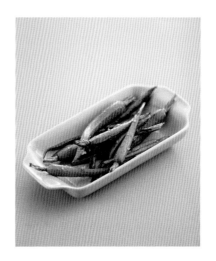

traffic-light mash

per serving 8.9g total fat
(5.4g saturated fat); 1455kJ
(348 cal); 48.8g carbohydrate;
13.2g protein; 9.1g fibre

Cook 1 chopped small kumara,
1 unpeeled small beetroot and
1½ cups frozen peas, separately,
until tender; drain, reserving
1 tablespoon cooking liquid. Peel
beetroot; process with reserved
cooking liquid until smooth; place in
small bowl. Mash peas and kumara,
separately, in small bowls. Cook
1kg chopped potato until tender;
drain. Mash potato; stir in ¾ cup
low-fat hot milk and 40g butter. Divide
potato among beetroot, pea and
kumara mash; mix well.

grilled corn and avocado salsa

per serving 15.2g total fat
(3.1g saturated fat); 1037kJ
(248 cal); 19.2g carbohydrate;
5.8g protein; 6.7g fibre

Cook 2 buttered corn cobs on heated
oiled grill plate (or grill or barbecue),
turning often, until browned. When
cool enough to handle, cut kernels
from cobs. Combine kernels in
medium bowl with 1 finely chopped
small red onion, 1 chopped large
avocado, 250g halved cherry
tomatoes, 2 thinly sliced green
onions, 1 tablespoon lime juice and
1 tablespoon sweet chilli sauce.

orange and maple carrots

per serving: 0.1g total fat
(0g saturated fat); 196kJ
(47 cal); 8.7g carbohydrate;
1.3g protein; 2.6g fibre

Preheat oven to 220°C/200°C
fan-forced. Combine 250g baby
carrots, 1 tablespoon maple syrup
and 1 tablespoon orange juice in
oiled medium baking dish; roast
10 minutes. Add 150g baby
green beans to dish; roast about
10 minutes or until vegetables are
tender. Stir in 1 teaspoon finely
grated orange rind.

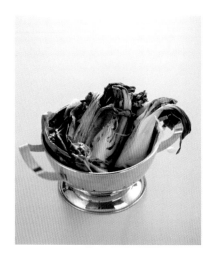
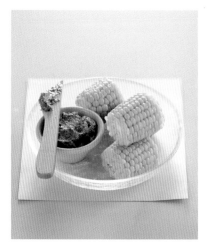

asian greens with soy dressing

per serving 1g total fat
(0.1g saturated fat); 150kJ
(36 cal); 2.5g carbohydrate;
2.9g protein; 2.8g fibre

Combine 2 tablespoons rice vinegar,
2 tablespoons light soy sauce,
½ teaspoon sesame oil and 2cm
piece finely chopped fresh ginger in
bowl. Cook 350g trimmed gai lan
and 500g trimmed and quartered
baby buk choy, separately, until
tender; drain. Serve greens drizzled
with soy dressing.

pesto corn cobs

per serving 14.1g total fat
(6.4g saturated fat); 1271kJ
(304 cal); 30.4g carbohydrate;
9.7g protein; 8.8g fibre

Blend or process 40g butter, 1 cup
chopped fresh basil, 1 quartered
clove garlic, 1 tablespoon roasted
pine nuts and 2 tablespoons grated
parmesan cheese until smooth.
Cover; refrigerate pesto until
required. Cut 4 large trimmed corn
cobs into quarters; boil, steam or
microwave until tender, drain. Serve
with pesto.

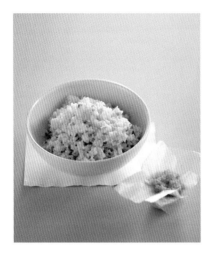

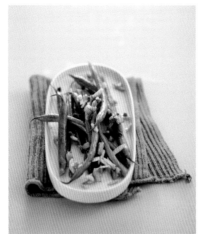

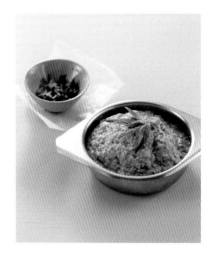

steamed lemon jasmine rice

per serving 4.8g total fat
(2.9g saturated fat); 957kJ
(229 cal); 41.3g carbohydrate;
4.5g protein; 1.5g fibre

Combine 1 cup jasmine rice,
20g butter, 1½ cups chicken stock
and ½ cup water in saucepan; bring
to a boil. Reduce heat; simmer,
covered tightly, about 10 minutes or
until rice is cooked. Remove from
heat; stand, covered, 5 minutes. Stir
in 2 teaspoons finely grated lemon
rind and ¼ cup chopped fresh chives.

green beans almondine

per serving 11.5g total fat
(3.9g saturated fat); 602kJ
(144 cal); 2.3g carbohydrate;
6.9g protein; 2.9g fibre

Cook 300g green beans until just
tender; drain. Rinse beans under
cold water; drain. Melt 20g butter
in large frying pan; cook 1 crushed
garlic clove, 1 finely chopped rindless
bacon rasher and ¼ cup slivered
almonds, stirring, until bacon crisps.
Add beans; stir until hot.

creamed mint peas

per serving 0.7g total fat
(0.1g saturated fat); 40kJ
(98 cal); 9.6g carbohydrate;
9.5g protein; 8g fibre

Cook 500g frozen peas and
2 unpeeled garlic cloves in saucepan
of boiling water until peas soften;
drain. Peel garlic; blend or process
with peas, ½ cup low-fat yogurt and
½ cup fresh mint leaves until smooth.

desserts

chocolate, pear and hazelnut parcels

preparation time 10 minutes
cooking time 30 minutes **serves** 4
per serving 7.5g total fat
(1g saturated fat); 1246kJ
(298 cal); 50.5g carbohydrate;
4.4g protein; 4.3g fibre

8 sheets fillo pastry
cooking-oil spray
4 medium pears (920g), peeled,
   cored, sliced thinly
1 tablespoon brown sugar
1 tablespoon chocolate-
   hazelnut spread

1 Preheat oven to 200°C/180°C fan-forced. Grease and line two oven trays.
2 Place two sheets of fillo on board; cover remaining sheets with baking paper then a damp tea towel to prevent it drying out. Spray uncovered pastry with cooking-oil spray. Place half of 1 sliced pear lengthways down centre of pastry; top with 1 teaspoon each of the sugar and the spread.
3 Fold in two long sides of pastry then roll from one narrow side to enclose filling. Place parcel, seam-side down, on tray. Repeat process with remaining pastry, pear, sugar and spread.
4 Spray parcels with cooking-oil spray. Bake about 10 minutes or until browned lightly. Serve with vanilla ice-cream if you like.

did you know? Children are born with an innate sweet preference, so it's no surprise that breast milk has a relatively high quantity of lactose or milk sugar. The key is to indulge this sweet tooth as your children grow, with naturally sweet, nutrient-rich foods like poached fruit.

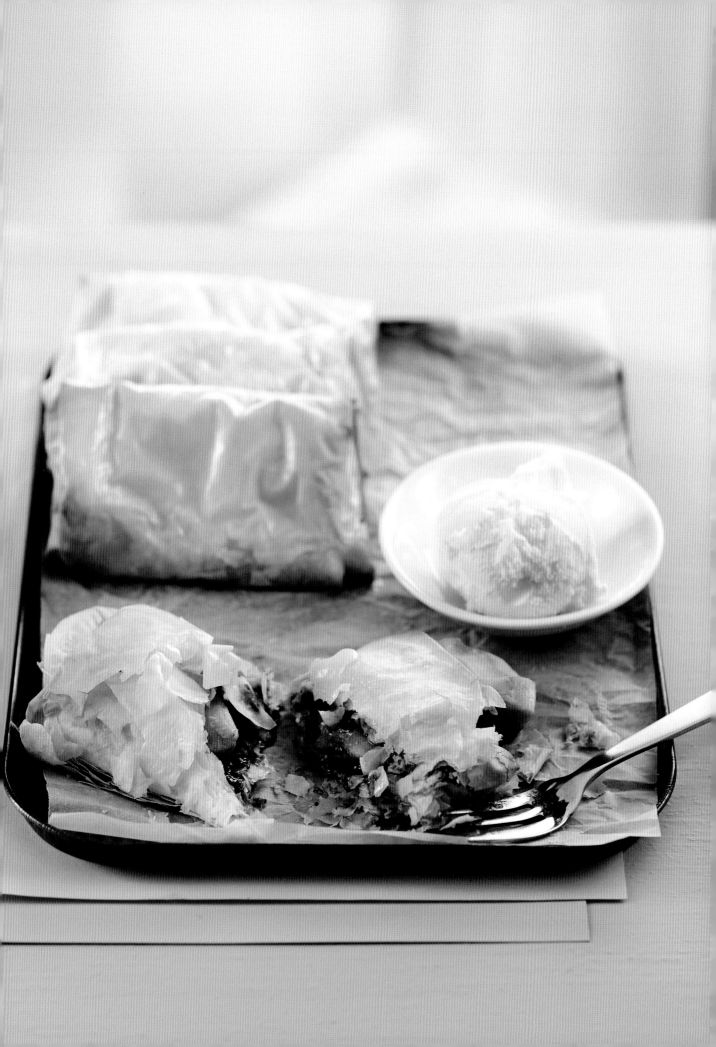

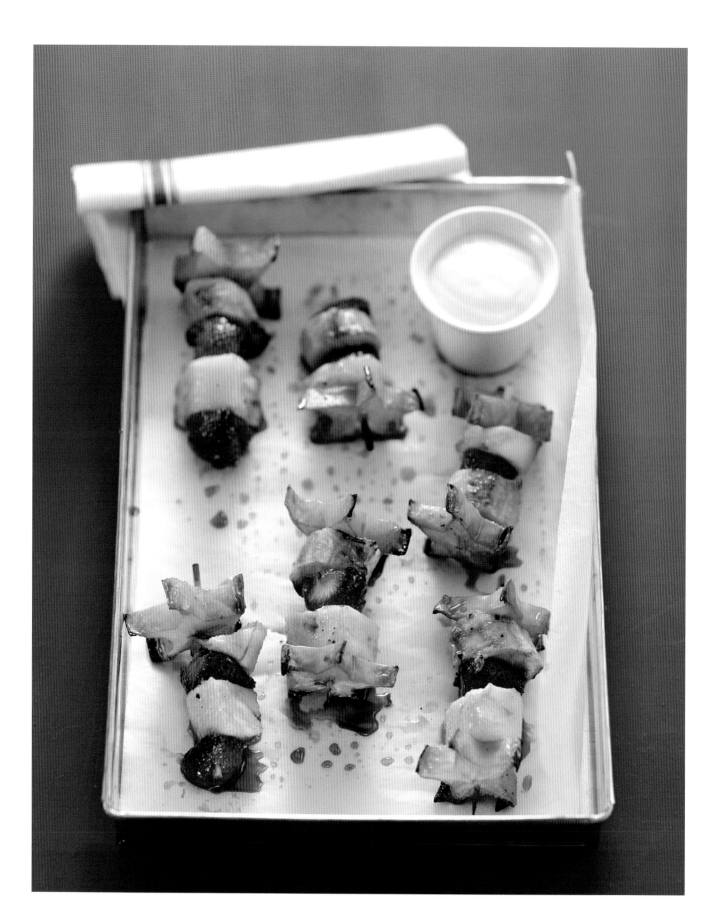

tropical fruit skewers with orange glaze

preparation time 20 minutes
cooking time 15 minutes **serves** 4
per serving 0.5g total fat
(0.1g saturated fat); 974kJ
(233 cal); 45.9g carbohydrate;
7.1g protein; 7.3g fibre

*You need about half a medium-sized
pineapple (1.25kg) for this recipe.
Soak eight 20cm-long wooden skewers
in water for one hour before using to
prevent them from splintering or
scorching during cooking.*

1 teaspoon finely grated orange rind
¼ cup (60ml) orange juice
2 tablespoons brown sugar
2 medium bananas (460g)
250g strawberries
600g piece pineapple
1 starfruit (160g)
200g low-fat vanilla yogurt

1 Combine rind, juice and sugar
in small saucepan; stir over low
heat until sugar dissolves. Cool.
2 Preheat grill.
3 Peel bananas; slice thickly
crossways. Hull and halve berries.
Peel pineapple; cut into chunks.
Slice starfruit thickly.
4 Thread fruits, alternately, onto
skewers. Place skewers on oven
tray lined with baking paper; pour
orange mixture over skewers, coating
all fruit pieces.
5 Grill skewers, turning occasionally,
about 10 minutes or until browned
lightly. Serve with yogurt.

did you know? Fruit juices can provide a range of vitamins and minerals, including vitamin C, folate, potassium and antioxidants. However, due to the concentrated natural fruit sugar (fructose), it's best to dilute juice with water, especially for young children.

upside-down cake with caramelised apple

preparation time 15 minutes
cooking time 25 minutes **serves** 8
per serving 10g total fat
(5.8g saturated fat); 970kJ
(232 cal); 28.9g carbohydrate;
4.9g protein; 1.7g fibre

2 large apples (400g)
60g unsalted butter, chopped
½ cup (110g) firmly packed
   brown sugar
1 teaspoon ground cinnamon
⅓ cup (50g) wholemeal
   self-raising flour
⅓ cup (80ml) low-fat milk
4 eggs, separated
¼ cup (55g) caster sugar
2 tablespoons flaked coconut

1 Preheat oven to 200°C/180°C fan-forced.
2 Peel and core apples; slice into 5mm rings.
3 Melt butter in heavy-based 25cm frying pan; add brown sugar and cinnamon; cook, stirring, until sugar dissolves. Remove from heat.
4 Place apple rings, overlapping slightly, on top of caramel in pan. Return to heat; cook, covered, over low heat, 2 minutes. Uncover; cook, over low heat, about 5 minutes or until apples are tender. Remove from heat.
5 Meanwhile, combine flour, milk and egg yolks in medium bowl.
6 Beat egg whites in small bowl with electric mixer until soft peaks form; gradually add caster sugar, beating until dissolved between additions. Fold egg white mixture into flour mixture, in two batches.
7 Spread mixture carefully over apple in pan. Bake, uncovered, in oven, about 12 minutes. Turn onto serving plate; serve sprinkled with coconut and, if you like, vanilla ice-cream.

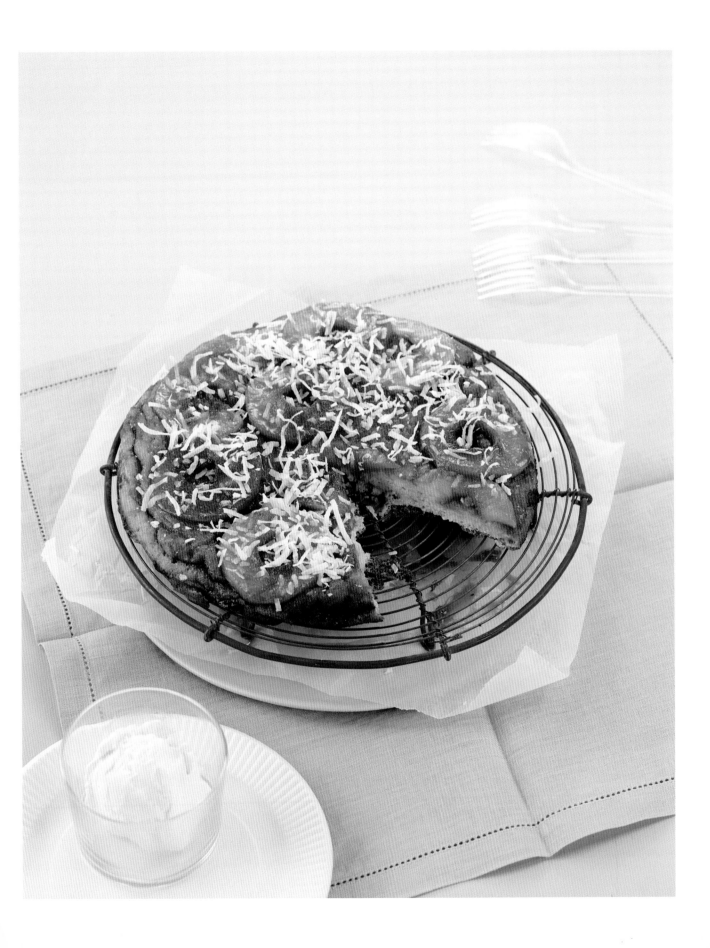

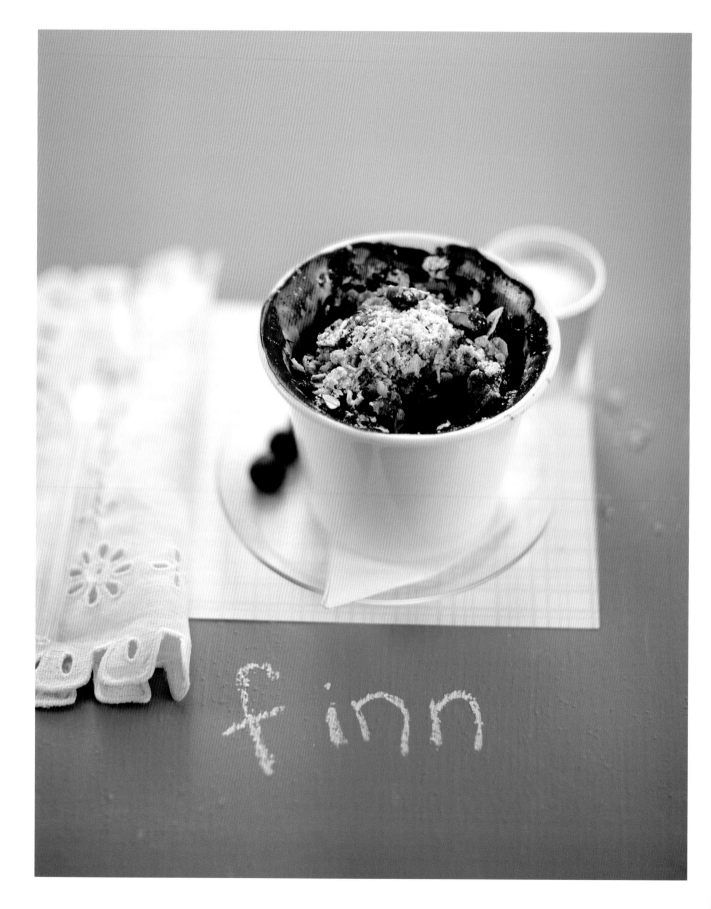

apple berry crumbles

preparation time 15 minutes
cooking time 30 minutes **serves** 4
per serving 9.3g total fat
(3g saturated fat); 8.3kJ
(192 cal); 22.3g carbohydrate;
3.1g protein; 3.1g fibre

2 medium apples (300g)
¾ cup (115g) frozen mixed berries
2 tablespoons lemon juice
2 tablespoons brown sugar
2 tablespoons plain flour
¼ cup (20g) rolled oats
20g butter
¼ cup (30g) finely chopped
   roasted hazelnuts

1 Preheat oven to 200°C/180°C fan-forced. Grease four ¾-cup (180ml) ovenproof dishes; place on oven tray.
2 Peel and core apples; chop coarsely. Combine apple, berries, juice and half the sugar in medium bowl; divide mixture among dishes.
3 Combine remaining sugar, flour and oats in small bowl. Rub butter into flour mixture; stir in nuts. Divide crumble over fruit mixture, pressing down firmly. Bake, uncovered, about 30 minutes or until browned lightly. Serve, if you like, dusted with icing sugar and accompanied with yogurt.

did you know? More and more childcare centres and schools are becoming nut-free zones to protect children with severe allergies. However, nuts are highly nutritious foods, packed with protein, vitamin E and healthy fats, so make sure you serve them at home. Finely chopped or crushed nuts and nut butters are best for children under five.

orange crème caramels

preparation time 20 minutes (plus refrigeration time)
cooking time 1 hour **makes** 6
per serving 3.8g total fat (1.8g saturated); 1170kJ (280 cal); 52.8g carbohydrate; 7.9g protein; 0.1g fibre

This dessert is pure bliss – creamy orange custard with a quintessential toffee topping.

1¼ cups (275g) caster sugar
½ cup (125ml) water
¼ cup (60ml) orange juice
2 cups (500ml) low-fat milk
3 eggs
3 egg yolks
1 teaspoon vanilla extract
2 teaspoons finely grated orange rind

1 Preheat oven to 160°C/140°C fan-forced.

2 Combine ¾ cup of the sugar with the water in medium heavy-based saucepan; stir over low heat, without boiling, until sugar dissolves. Bring to a boil; boil, uncovered, without stirring, until mixture is caramel in colour. Remove from heat; add juice (some of the toffee will set; stir over low heat until toffee melts). Divide mixture among six ½-cup (125ml) ovenproof dishes.

3 Bring milk to a boil in small saucepan. Whisk remaining sugar, eggs, egg yolks and extract in medium bowl; whisk hot milk gradually into egg mixture. Stir in the rind; pour mixture over toffee in dishes.

4 Place dishes in medium baking dish; add enough boiling water to come halfway up the sides of dishes. Bake about 45 minutes or until custards set. Remove dishes from baking dish, cool 10 minutes then cover; refrigerate overnight.

5 Using fingers, gently ease each custard away from side of dish then invert onto individual serving plates.

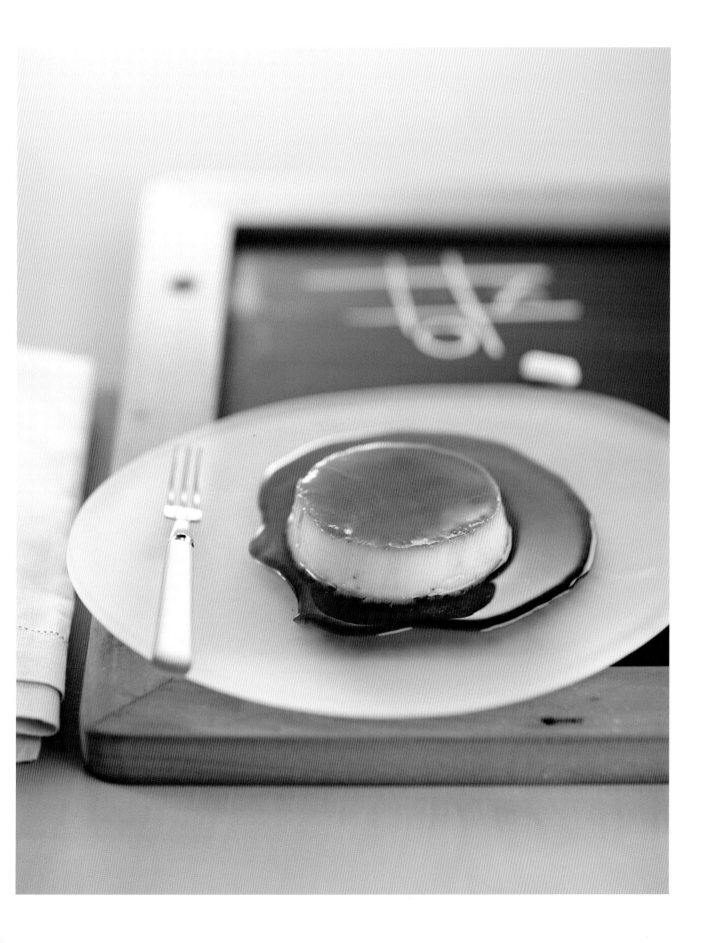

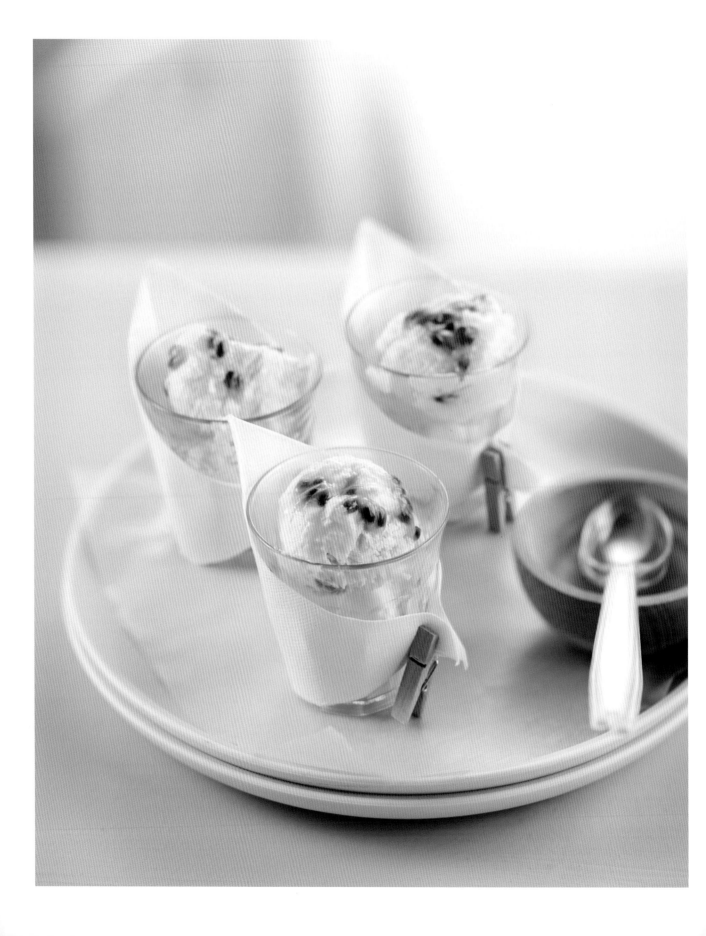

frozen green apple yogurt

preparation time 15 minutes
(plus freezing time)
cooking time 5 minutes **serves** 4
per serving 4.3g total fat
(2.8g saturated fat); 903kJ
(216 cal); 36.8g carbohydrate;
6.7g protein; 0.7g fibre

*Refreshing frozen yogurt certainly
gives ice-cream a run for its money.
You need to buy an apple weighing
about 275g for this recipe.*

⅓ cup (115g) honey
½ cup (125ml) apple juice
1 teaspoon gelatine
¾ cup (130g) finely grated
    unpeeled apple
500g greek-style yogurt

1 Stir honey and juice in small
saucepan over low heat until
honey melts; cool syrup 5 minutes.
2 Sprinkle gelatine over syrup; stir
until gelatine dissolves.
3 Combine gelatine mixture, apple
and yogurt in 14cm x 21cm loaf pan.
Cover with foil; freeze 3 hours or
overnight. Remove yogurt from freezer
about 15 minutes before serving.

variations
raspberry
Substitute water for the juice in
syrup; substitute 150g thawed frozen
raspberries for the apple. Push
thawed raspberries through a fine
sieve over small bowl; discard seeds.
per serving 4.4g total fat
(2.8g saturated fat); 840kJ
(201 cal); 31.7g carbohydrate;
7.1g protein; 2g fibre

mango
Substitute water for the juice in syrup;
substitute 300g thawed coarsely
chopped frozen mango for the apple.
per serving 4.4g total fat
(2.8g saturated fat); 957kJ
(229 cal); 38.9g carbohydrate;
4.4g protein; 1.1g fibre

did you know? Many yogurts contain beneficial bacteria known as live active cultures that help boost the levels of good bacteria in your child's gut. Research shows that probiotic yogurts can help your child recover from a bout of gastroenteritis.

rice pudding with blueberry compote

preparation time 10 minutes
cooking time 1 hour 15 minutes
serves 4
per serving 0.6g total fat
(0.2g saturated fat); 1175kJ
(280 cal); 56.3g carbohydrate;
10.9g protein; 1.5g fibre

You can use any type of berry you like in the compote.

½ cup (100g) calrose rice
3 cups (750ml) low-fat milk
1 teaspoon vanilla extract
¼ cup (55g) caster sugar
1⅓ cups (200g) fresh or
    frozen blueberries
1 tablespoon caster sugar, extra

1 Preheat oven to 180°C/160°C fan-forced.
2 Rinse rice under cold water; drain, spread into shallow 1.5-litre (6-cup) ovenproof dish.
3 Bring milk, extract and sugar to a boil in medium saucepan then pour over rice. Bake, covered, about 1 hour 10 minutes or until rice softens and liquid is absorbed.
4 Meanwhile, combine blueberries and extra sugar in small saucepan; stir over low heat until sugar dissolves. Cool 10 minutes.
5 Serve compote with pudding.

fruit salad and yogurt trifle

preparation time 25 minutes
(plus refrigeration time) serves 8
per serving 7.1g total fat
(4.2g saturated fat); 1129kJ
(270 cal); 46.4g carbohydrate;
8.7g protein; 4.5g fibre

The goodness of fruit salad with a special touch of jam rollettes and jelly: this layered delight is healthy and scrummy in one hit. Jam rollettes (mini swiss-rolls) are available in most supermarkets.
You need to buy three passionfruits for this recipe.

85g packet raspberry jelly crystals
1 cup (135g) fresh or
    frozen raspberries
6 x 30g jam rollettes, sliced thickly
250g strawberries, quartered
1 small orange (180g), segmented
2 medium kiwifruits (170g), peeled,
    chopped coarsely
¼ cup (60ml) passionfruit pulp
250g reduced-fat
    cream cheese, softened
1 tablespoon icing sugar
1½ cups (420g) low-fat
    mixed berry yogurt
1 starfruit (160g), cut into 8 slices

1 Make jelly according to directions on packet; divide among eight 1-cup (250ml) serving glasses, sprinkle with raspberries. Cover; refrigerate 3 hours or until jelly is firm.
2 Top jelly with rollette slices then strawberries, orange, kiwifruit and passionfruit pulp.
3 Beat cream cheese and icing sugar in small bowl with electric mixer until smooth. Gradually beat in yogurt; spread mixture over fruit in glasses. Cover trifles; refrigerate 1 hour. Top with starfruit to serve.

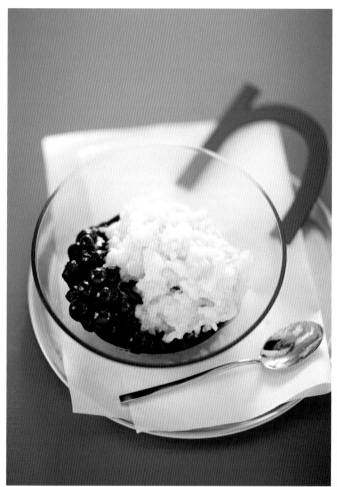

rice pudding with blueberry compote

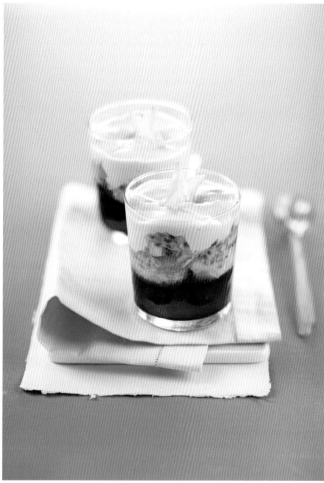

fruit salad and yogurt trifle

baking

yogurt, berry and white chocolate muffins

preparation time 10 minutes
cooking time 25 minutes **makes** 12
per muffin 7.2g total fat
(2.5g saturated fat); 807kJ
(193 cal); 25.3g carbohydrate;
5.6g protein; 2.4g fibre

You can use milk or dark chocolate instead of white for the muffins and still get the same melt-in-the-mouth result. These muffins are best served warm.

1½ cups (225g) wholemeal
  self-raising flour
½ cup (110g) caster sugar
2 tablespoons vegetable oil
2 eggs, beaten lightly
1 cup (280g) low-fat yogurt
1 cup (150g) frozen mixed berries
100g white eating chocolate,
  chopped coarsely

1 Preheat oven to 180°C/160°C fan-forced. Grease 12-hole (⅓-cup/80ml) muffin pan.
2 Combine flour and sugar in large bowl. Add remaining ingredients; mix batter until just combined. Divide batter among pan holes. Bake about 30 minutes. Stand muffins 5 minutes before serving, dusted with sifted icing sugar, if you like.

did you know? Research shows that probiotic yogurts can help boost immunity. So look for yogurts with the letters "ABC" or words like "probiotics" or "live active cultures" when shopping.

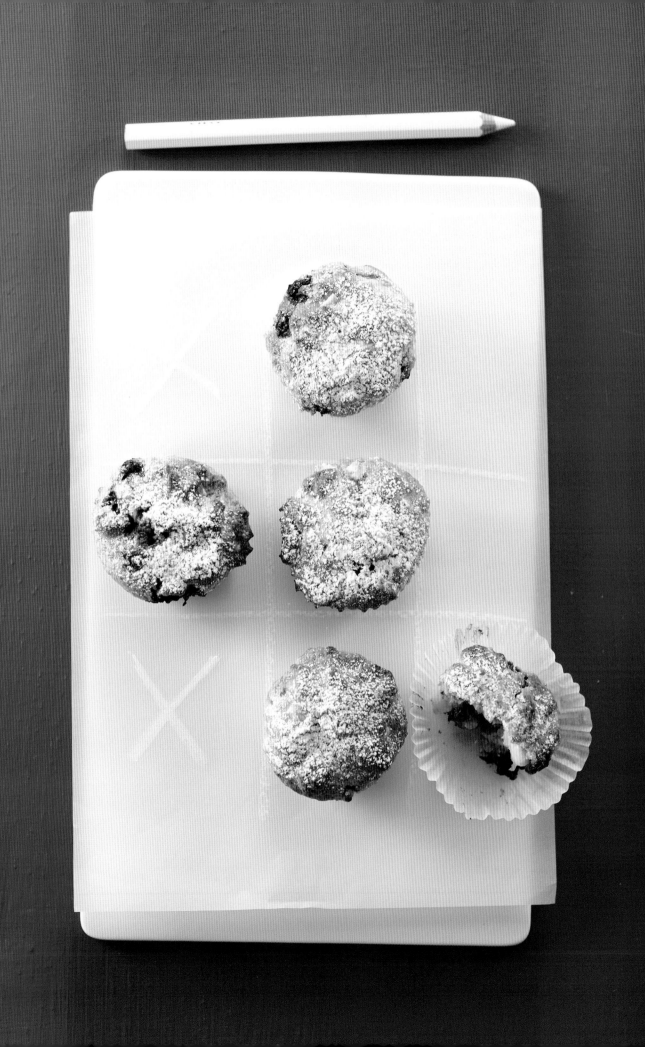

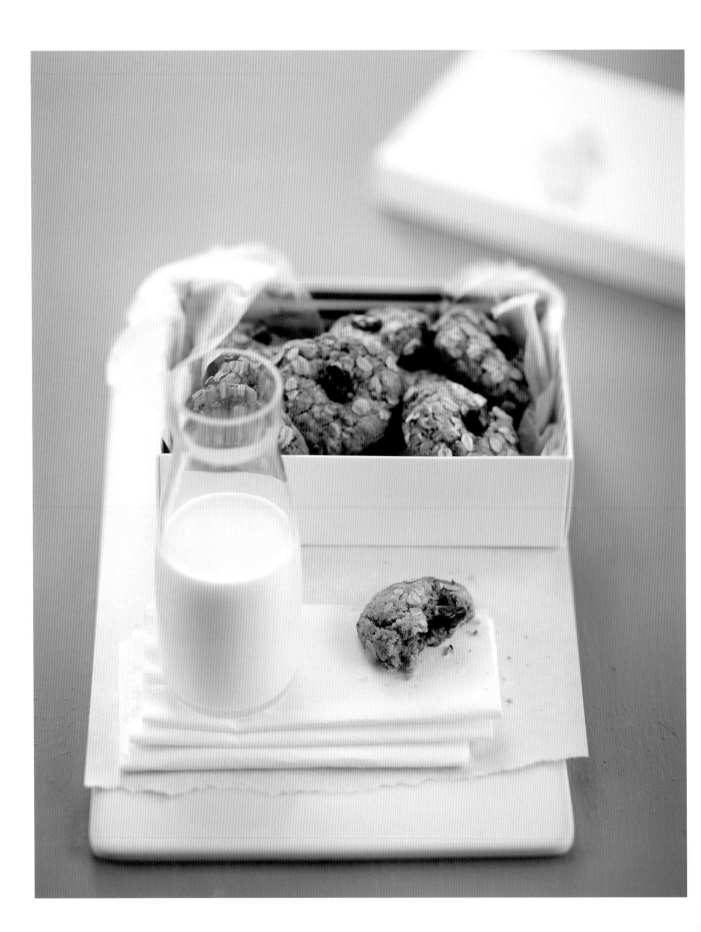

banana, date and rolled oat cookies

preparation time 20 minutes
cooking time 15 minutes makes 28
per cookie 4.4g total fat
(2.6g saturated fat); 539kJ
(129 cal); 19.9g carbohydrate;
1.7g protein; 1.7g fibre

*You need one medium overripe
banana (230g) for this recipe.*

125g butter, softened
1 teaspoon finely grated lemon rind
1 cup (220g) firmly packed
   brown sugar
1 egg yolk
⅓ cup mashed banana
1½ cups (225g) plain flour
½ teaspoon bicarbonate of soda
1 cup (90g) rolled oats
½ cup (75g) finely chopped
   dried dates
⅔ cup (60g) rolled oats, extra
4 dried dates (35g), seeded,
   chopped coarsely

1 Preheat oven to 180°C/160°C fan-forced. Grease oven trays; line with baking paper.
2 Beat butter, rind, sugar and egg yolk in small bowl with electric mixer until combined; stir in banana then sifted flour and soda, oats and dates.
3 Roll level tablespoons of mixture into balls; roll each ball in extra oats then place on trays 5cm apart. Press a piece of coarsely chopped date into centre of each ball. Bake about 15 minutes. Cool cookies on trays.

did you know? Many commercial cakes and biscuits are labelled with "traces of nuts" as they may be manufactured next to products with nuts. So, if you have friends or family members with nut allergies, the best approach is home baking, so you have final control over what you add.

hummingbird cupcakes

preparation time 20 minutes
cooking time 25 minutes **makes** 12
per cupcake 9.1g total fat
(2.6g saturated fat); 1195kJ
(286 cal); 45.4g carbohydrate;
4.1g protein; 2.4g fibre

You need two medium overripe bananas (460g) for this recipe.

440g can crushed pineapple
  in syrup
1 cup (160g) wholemeal plain flour
½ cup (80g) wholemeal
  self-raising flour
½ teaspoon bicarbonate of soda
½ teaspoon ground cinnamon
½ teaspoon ground ginger
1 cup (220g) firmly packed
  brown sugar
2 eggs, beaten lightly
¼ cup (20g) desiccated coconut
¾ cup mashed banana
⅓ cup (80ml) vegetable oil
½ cup (80g) icing sugar
2 tablespoons toasted
  shredded coconut

1 Preheat oven to 180°C/160°C fan-forced. Line 12-hole (⅓-cup/80ml) muffin pan with paper cases.

2 Drain pineapple over small bowl, pressing with spoon to extract as much syrup as possible. Reserve ⅓ cup of the syrup, discard remainder.

3 Sift flours, soda, spices and brown sugar into medium bowl. Stir in ¼ cup of the reserved syrup, egg, desiccated coconut, banana and oil; divide mixture among pan holes.

4 Bake about 25 minutes. Stand 5 minutes; turn, top-side up, onto wire rack to cool.

5 Meanwhile, place icing sugar in small bowl; add enough of the remaining syrup to make icing spreadable. Drizzle cupcakes with icing, sprinkle with shredded coconut.

did you know? Canned fruit can count towards your child's daily fruit serves. Fruit snack packs are a great, go anywhere snack. You can also top yogurt or ice-cream with canned peaches, pears, plums, apricots, cherries or pineapple.

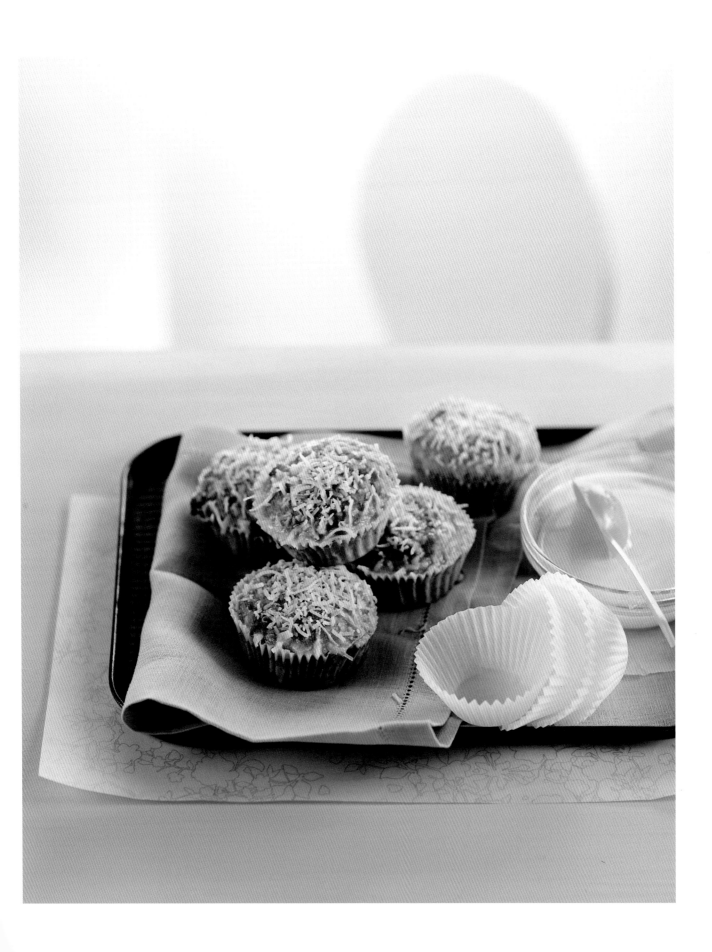

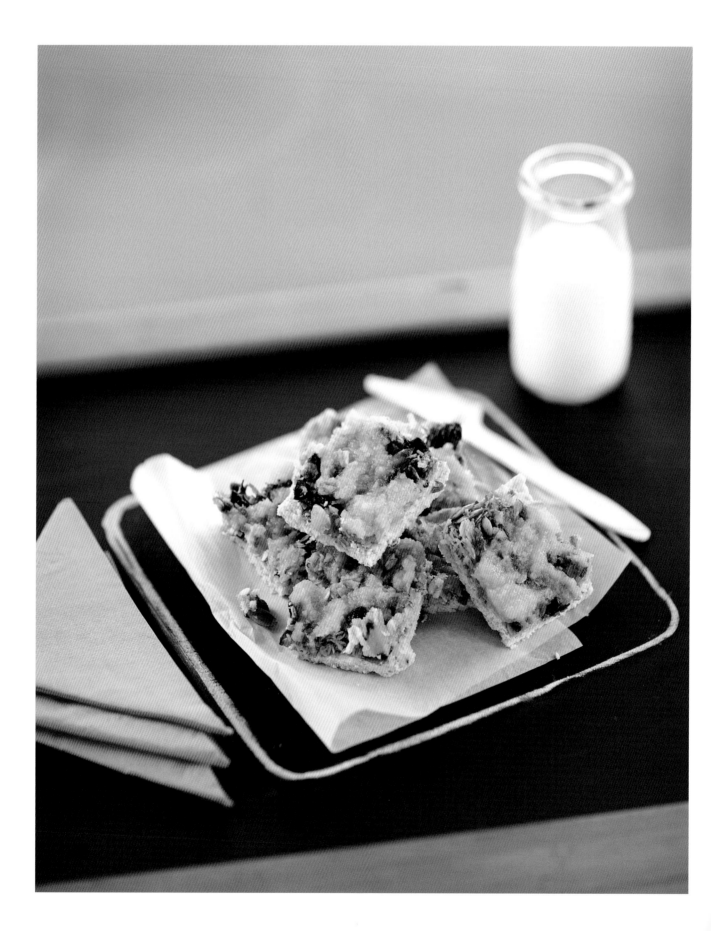

fruit muesli slice

preparation time 25 minutes
(plus referigeration time)
cooking time 25 minutes **makes** 20
per slice 6.7g total fat
(3.6g saturated fat); 627kJ
(150 cal); 19.8g carbohydrate;
1.7g protein; 1.8g fibre

2 tablespoons honey
100g butter, softened
⅓ cup (50g) finely chopped
    dried dates
¼ cup (60g) pepitas
1 cup (90g) rolled oats
⅓ cup (25g) shredded coconut
⅔ cup (100g) finely chopped
    dried apricots
½ cup (110g) caster sugar
1 egg yolk
⅔ cup (100g) plain flour
¼ cup (35g) self-raising flour
1 tablespoon custard powder
⅓ cup (80ml) hot water

1 Preheat oven to 180°C/160°C fan-forced. Grease 20cm x 30cm lamington pan; line with baking paper.
2 To make muesli, heat honey and a quarter of the butter in small saucepan, stirring until smooth. Transfer to medium bowl; stir in dates, pepitas, oats, coconut and half the apricots.
3 Beat sugar, egg yolk and remaining butter in small bowl with electric mixer until light and fluffy. Mix in sifted flours and custard powder. Press mixture over base of pan; sprinkle with muesli. Bake about 25 minutes.
4 Meanwhile, combine remaining apricots and the water in small saucepan; cook, stirring, about 10 minutes or until soft. Cool slightly; process mixture until smooth. Spread slice with apricot mixture; cool 10 minutes in pan then refrigerate 1 hour before cutting.

did you know? Pepitas are actually prepared pumpkin seeds that can be purchased plain or roasted and salted. Like nuts, they are high in protein and can be added to salads, baking or simply used for snacking.

banana loaf

preparation time 10 minutes
cooking time 40 minutes **serves** 12
per serving 2.1g total fat
(1.1g saturated fat); 698kJ
(167 cal); 32.5g carbohydrate;
3.1g protein; 1.9g fibre

*You need to mash one large overripe
banana (230g) for this recipe.*

¾ cup (120g) wholemeal
    self-raising flour
½ cup (75g) self-raising flour
1 teaspoon ground cinnamon
20g butter
½ cup (110g) firmly packed
    brown sugar
1 egg
¼ cup (60ml) low-fat milk
½ cup mashed banana
⅓ cup (115g) honey
2 small bananas (260g),
    sliced thickly

1 Preheat oven to 200°C/180°C
fan-forced. Grease 8cm x 26cm bar
cake pan; line base with baking paper.
2 Process flours, cinnamon and
butter until crumbly. Add sugar, egg,
milk and mashed banana; pulse until
ingredients are just combined. Pour
mixture into pan.
3 Bake about 40 minutes. Stand
loaf 5 minutes; turn, top-side up,
onto wire rack to cool. Serve sliced,
topped with honey and sliced banana.

did you know? Bananas are rich in fibre, including a special type of fibre known as resistant starch that is important for bowel health. Green or firm bananas are higher in resistant starch than ripe bananas.

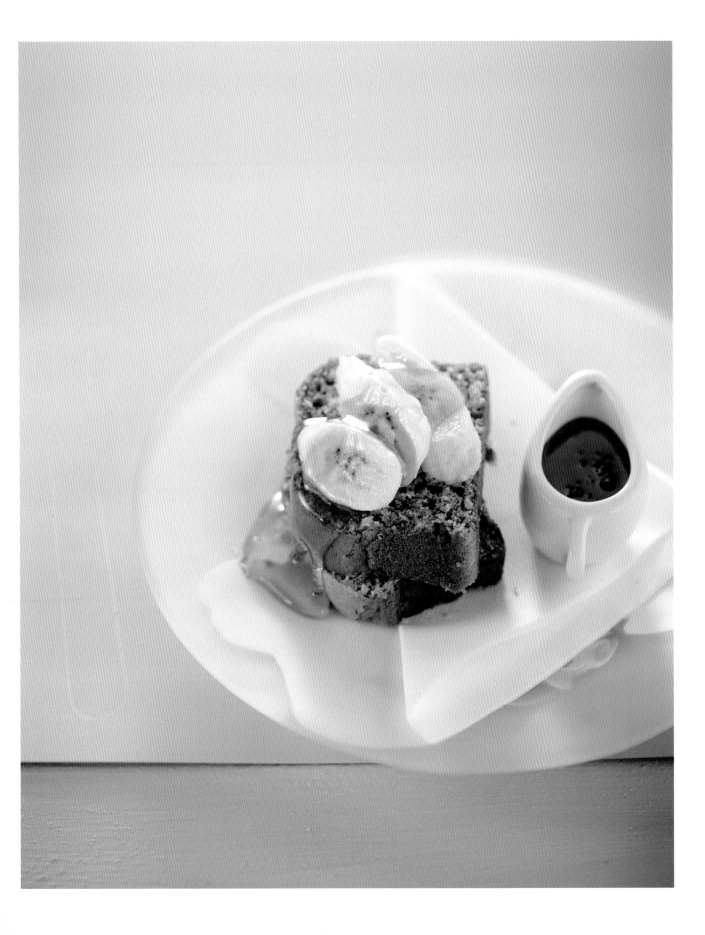

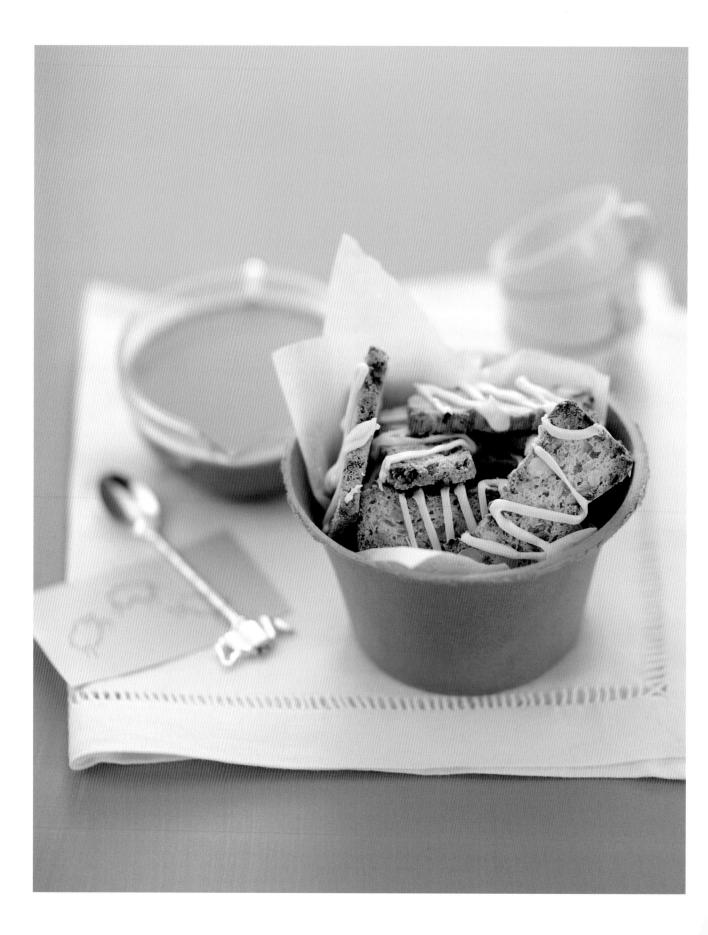

white choc, apple and almond biscuits

preparation time 10 minutes
(plus cooling time)
cooking time 1 hour **makes** 50
per biscuit 1.6g total fat
(0.3g saturated fat); 155kJ
(37 cal); 4.4g carbohydrate;
1g protein; 0.4g fibre

*Our new version of the classic Italian
creation, biscotti, is sure to be a hit.
These biscuits will keep, stored in an
airtight container, at a cool room
temperature for at least a month.*

3 egg whites
⅓ cup (75g) caster sugar
¾ cup (110g) plain flour
¼ teaspoon ground cinnamon
⅔ cup (110g) whole
    blanched almonds
1 cup (55g) finely chopped
    dried apples
50g white eating chocolate, melted

1 Preheat oven to 180°C/160°C
fan-forced. Grease 8cm x 26cm bar
cake pan; line base with baking
paper, extending paper 5cm over
long sides.
2 Beat egg whites and sugar in
small bowl with electric mixer until
sugar dissolves. Fold in sifted flour
then cinnamon, nuts and apple;
spread into pan.
3 Bake about 30 minutes. Stand
10 minutes; turn, top-side up, onto
wire rack to cool.
4 Reduce oven temperature to
150°C/130°C fan-forced.
5 Using serrated knife, slice cooled
bread thinly; place slices on oven
trays. Bake about 15 minutes or until
crisp. Turn onto wire rack to cool.
Drizzle biscuits with chocolate.

strawberry jelly cakes

preparation time 45 minutes (plus refrigeration time)
cooking time 25 minutes **makes** 36
per cake 6.7g total fat (5g saturated fat); 456kJ (109 cal); 10.2g carbohydrate; 1g protein; 1.2g fibre

You need 2 large passionfruits for this recipe.
Jelly cakes will keep, stored in an airtight container in the refrigerator, for up to one week.

125g butter, softened
½ teaspoon vanilla extract
½ cup (110g) caster sugar
2 eggs
1½ cups (225g) self-raising flour
⅓ cup (80ml) low-fat milk
1¾ cups (430ml) boiling water
85g packet strawberry jelly crystals
2 tablespoons passionfruit pulp
1½ cups (75g) flaked coconut
1½ cups (115g) shredded coconut

1 Preheat oven to 180°C/160°C fan-forced. Grease deep 23cm-square cake pan; line base with baking paper.
2 Beat butter, extract and sugar in small bowl with electric mixer until light and fluffy. Beat in eggs, one at a time, until just combined. Stir in flour and milk until smooth; spread mixture into pan.
3 Bake about 25 minutes. Stand 5 minutes; turn, top-side up, onto wire rack to cool.
4 Meanwhile, stir the water and jelly in medium heatproof jug until crystals dissolve; stir pulp into jelly. Pour into 19cm x 29cm slice pan; refrigerate, stirring occasionally, until set to the consistency of unbeaten egg white.
5 Cut cake into 36 squares; dip each square into jelly then combined coconuts. Cover jelly cakes on tray; refrigerate 30 minutes.

did you know? That great Aussie backyard favourite, passionfruit, is also a winner with kids. Due to the edible seeds, passionfruit is one of the highest fruit sources of dietary fibre.

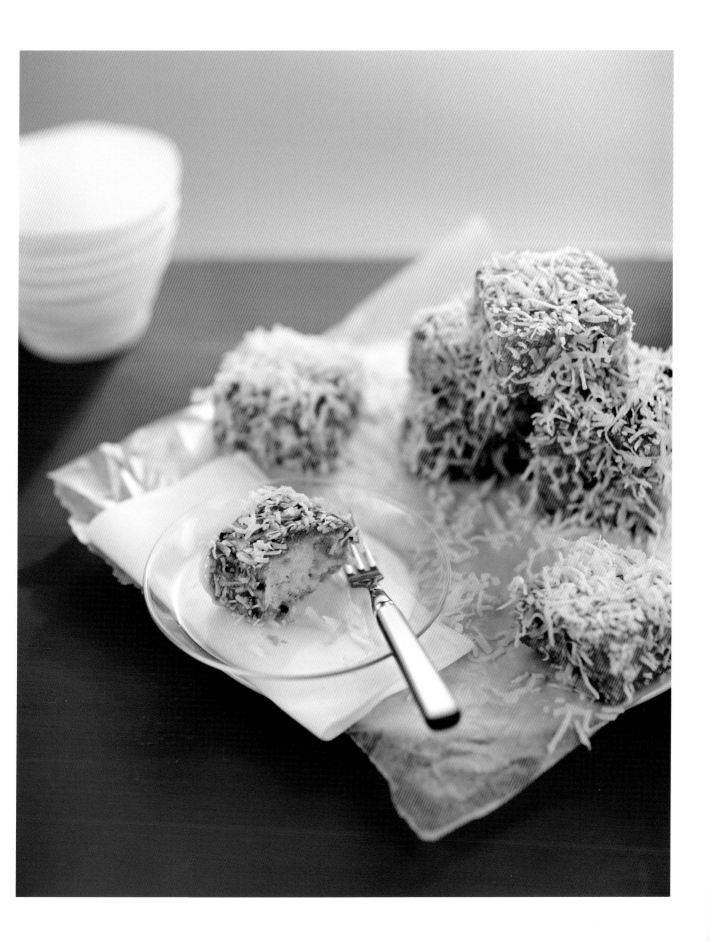

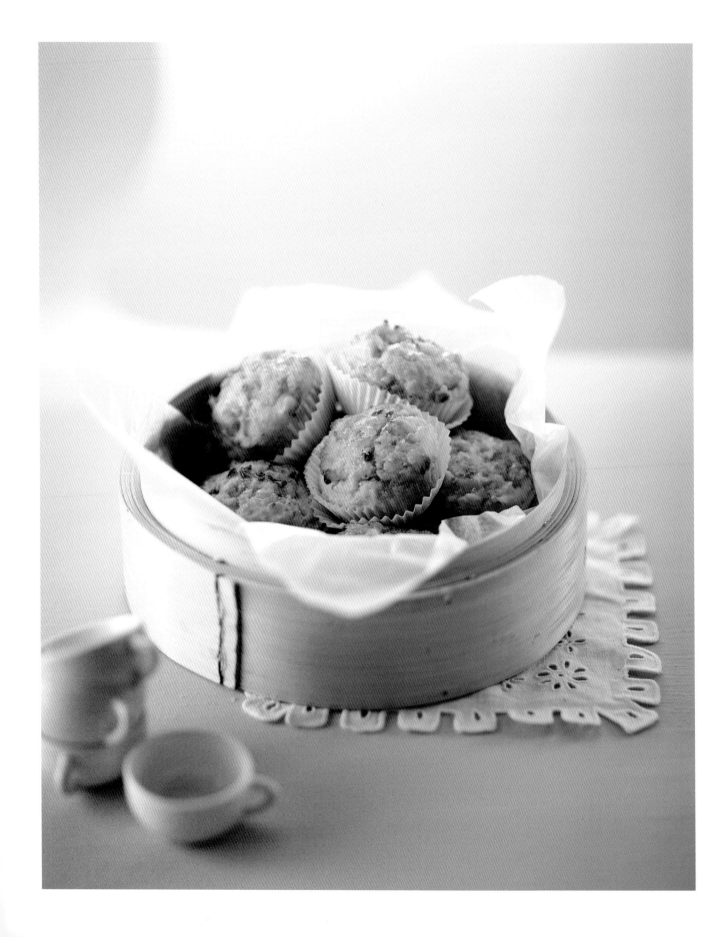

cream cheese, corn and sweet chilli muffins

preparation time 10 minutes (plus standing time)
cooking time 20 minutes **makes** 12
per muffin 6.4g total fat (3.5g saturated fat); 786kJ (188 cal); 25.4g carbohydrate; 6.3g protein; 1.7g fibre

The smell of these muffins as they come out of the oven will whet any kid's appetite. Reheat leftover muffins in a microwave oven on HIGH (100%) for 20 seconds each.

½ cup (85g) polenta
1 cup (250ml) buttermilk
40g butter, melted
2 eggs, beaten lightly
⅓ cup (80ml) sweet chilli sauce
1 medium brown onion (150g), chopped finely
1½ cups (225g) self-raising flour
310g can corn kernels, drained
125g packet reduced-fat cream cheese

1 Preheat oven to 200°C/180°C fan-forced. Oil 12-hole (⅓-cup/80ml) muffin pan.

2 Mix polenta and buttermilk in small bowl; stand 20 minutes. Stir in butter, egg and two tablespoons of the sauce.

3 Meanwhile, cook onion in heated small frying pan, stirring, about 5 minutes or until onion softens. Cool 5 minutes.

4 Combine onion, flour and kernels in medium bowl. Add polenta mixture; mix batter until combined.

5 Spoon 1 tablespoon batter into each pan hole. Cut cheese into 12 equal pieces; place one piece into batter in pan then cover each with remaining batter, drizzle with remaining sauce.

6 Bake about 20 minutes. Serve muffins warm.

caramel banana pinwheels

preparation time 20 minutes
cooking time 30 minutes **makes** 10
per pinwheel 4.5g total fat
(1.6g saturated fat); 786kJ
(188 cal); 31g carbohydrate;
4.2g protein; 2.6g fibre

Home-baked treats can be healthier and more tasty than store-bought, and the kids can be involved in their making.

½ cup (110g) firmly packed
 brown sugar
1 cup (150g) self-raising flour
1 cup (160g) wholemeal
 self-raising flour
30g butter
3 small ripe bananas (390g)
½ cup (125ml) low-fat milk
⅓ cup (35g) finely
 chopped walnuts

1 Preheat oven to 200°C/180°C fan-forced. Grease 20cm-round sandwich pan; sprinkle base of pan with 2 tablespoons of the sugar.
2 Place flours and 1 tablespoon of the remaining sugar in medium bowl; rub in butter. Mash 1 of the bananas, add to bowl with milk; mix to a soft, sticky dough. Knead dough on floured surface; roll dough to 30cm x 40cm shape.
3 Chop remaining bananas finely. Sprinkle remaining sugar over dough, top with nuts and extra banana.
4 Starting from long side, roll dough tightly; trim ends. Cut roll into 10 slices; place pinwheels, cut-side up, in single layer, in pan. Bake about 30 minutes. Serve pinwheels warm.

ham and cheese pinwheels

preparation time 25 minutes
cooking time 35 minutes **makes** 12
per pinwheel 7.5g total fat
(3.9g saturated fat); 865kJ
(207 cal); 20.8g carbohydrate;
12.3g protein; 1.2g fibre

6 eggs, beaten lightly
2 cups (300g) self-raising flour
1 tablespoon caster sugar
30g butter
¾ cup (180ml) low-fat milk
¼ cup (70g) tomato paste
175g shaved ham, cut into
 thin strips
1 cup (120g) coarsely grated
 reduced-fat cheddar cheese

1 Preheat oven to 200°C/180°C fan-forced. Oil 19cm x 29cm slice pan.
2 Cook egg in oiled medium frying pan over low heat, stirring constantly, until scrambled.
3 Sift flour and sugar into medium bowl; rub in butter. Stir in milk; mix to a soft, sticky dough. Knead dough on floured surface; roll dough to 30cm x 40cm shape.
4 Spread tomato paste over dough; sprinkle with ham, top with egg then sprinkle with cheese.
5 Starting from long side, roll dough firmly; trim ends. Cut roll into 12 slices; place pinwheels, cut-side up, in single layer, in pan. Bake about 30 minutes. Serve pinwheels warm.

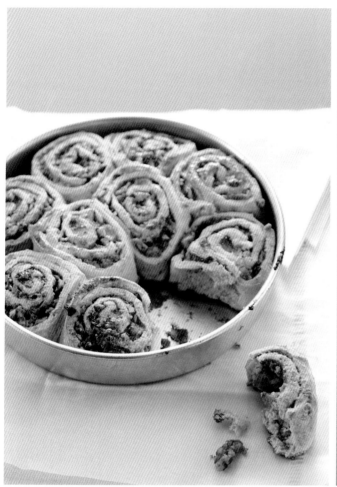

caramel banana pinwheels

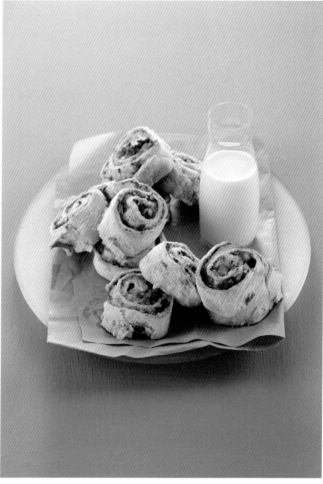

ham and cheese pinwheels

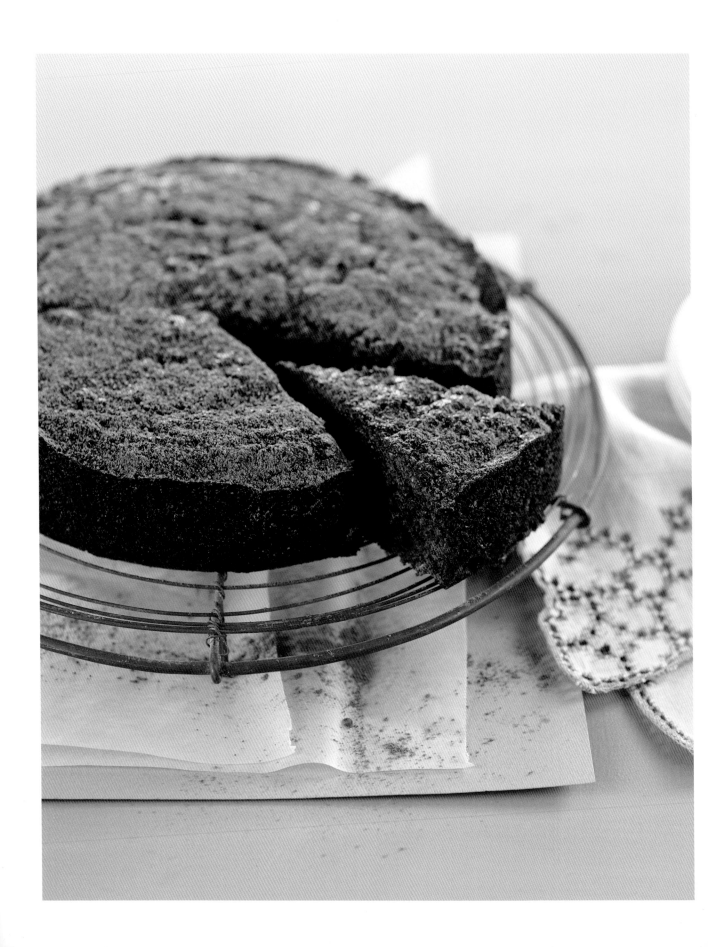

prune and choc-chip cake

preparation time 15 minutes
cooking time 1 hour **serves** 8
per serving 10.1g total fat
(6.1g saturated fat); 1292kJ
(309 cal); 48.3g carbohydrate;
3.7g protein; 4.4g fibre

1¼ cups (210g) seeded prunes
1¼ cups (310ml) boiling water
1 teaspoon bicarbonate of soda
60g butter, chopped
¾ cup (165g) firmly packed
   brown sugar
1 cup (160g) wholemeal
   self-raising flour
2 eggs
½ cup (95g) milk Choc Bits

1 Preheat oven to 180°C/160°C
fan-forced. Grease deep 20cm-round
cake pan; line base with baking paper.
2 Process prunes, the water and
soda until combined; stand, covered,
5 minutes.
3 Add butter and sugar to processor;
pulse until ingredients are combined.
Add flour and eggs; pulse until
combined. Stir in Choc Bits; pour
mixture into pan.
4 Bake about 1 hour. Stand cake
5 minutes; turn, top-side up, onto
wire rack to cool. Sprinkle with sifted
icing sugar, if you like.

did you know? Chocolate contains a host of naturally-occurring compounds that may explain its feel-good factor, but the surprising finding is that it also contains heart-friendly fats and antioxidants. Dark chocolate is higher in antioxidants than milk, so encourage your children to trial a taste for dark chocolate as they get older.

glossary

almonds, slivered small pieces cut lengthways.

beans

borlotti also known as roman beans or pink beans; can be eaten fresh or dried.

kidney medium-size red bean, slightly floury in texture yet sweet in flavour; sold dried or canned, it's found in bean mixes and is the bean used in chile con carne.

bicarbonate of soda also known as baking soda; a mild alkali used as a leavening agent in baking.

breads

lavash flat, unleavened bread of Mediterranean origin; good used as a wrapper or torn and used for dips.

pitta also known as lebanese bread; wheat-flour pocket bread sold in large, flat pieces that separate into two thin rounds. Also available in small thick pieces known as pocket pitta.

tortillas thin, round unleavened bread originating in Mexico; can be made of corn or wheat flour. Available in many sizes, they can be purchased frozen, fresh or vacuum-packed.

turkish sold in long (about 45cm) flat loaves as well as individual rounds; made from wheat flour and sprinkled with black onion seeds.

buk choy also known as bak choy, pak choi, chinese white cabbage or chinese chard; has a fresh, mild mustard taste. Use both stems and leaves.

baby buk choy, also known as pak kat farang or shanghai bok choy, is much smaller and more tender than buk choy. It has a mildly acrid taste.

cheese

bocconcini from the diminutive of "boccone", meaning mouthful in Italian; walnut-sized, baby mozzarella, a delicate, semi-soft, white cheese traditionally made from buffalo milk.

cheddar most common cow-milk tasty cheese; should be aged, hard and have a pronounced bite.

cream commonly known as philly or philadelphia; a soft cow-milk cheese.

fetta Greek in origin; a crumbly textured goat- or sheep-milk cheese having a sharp, salty taste. Ripened and stored in salted whey.

jarlsberg brand-name of a popular Norwegian cheese made from cow milk; has large holes and a mild, nutty taste.

pizza a commercial blend of varying proportions of processed grated mozzarella, cheddar and parmesan cheeses.

ricotta a soft, sweet, moist, white cow-milk cheese with a low fat content and a slightly grainy texture.

chocolate

milk Choc Bits also known as chocolate chips or chocolate morsels. Made of cocoa liquor, cocoa butter, sugar and an emulsifier. These hold their shape in baking and are ideal for decorating.

white eating contains no cocoa solids but derives its sweet flavour from cocoa butter. Very sensitive to heat.

coconut

desiccated concentrated, dried, unsweetened and finely shredded coconut flesh.

flaked dried flaked coconut flesh.

shredded unsweetened thin strips of dried coconut flesh.

couscous a fine, grain-like cereal product made from semolina; from the countries of North Africa.

cornflake crumbs a prepared finely ground mixture used for coating or crumbing food before frying or baking.

flour

buckwheat made from a herb in the same plant family as rhubarb; not a cereal, so it is gluten-free.

wholemeal, self-raising also known as wholewheat; milled with the wheat germ so is higher in fibre and more nutritional than plain flour.

gai lan also known as gai larn, chinese broccoli and chinese kale; a green vegetable appreciated more for its stems than its coarse leaves. Gai lan can be served steamed and stir-fried, in soups and noodle dishes. One of the most popular Asian greens.

gelatine a thickening agent. Available in sheet form, known as leaf gelatine or as a powder. Three teaspoons of dried gelatine (8g or one sachet) is roughly equivalent to four gelatine leaves.

kecap manis *see sauces.*

kumara the Polynesian name of an orange-fleshed sweet potato often confused with yam; good baked, boiled, mashed or fried similarly to other potatoes.

lebanese cucumber short, slender and thin-skinned. Probably the most popular variety because of its tender, edible skin, tiny yielding seeds, and sweet, fresh and flavoursome taste.

leek a member of the onion family, the leek resembles a green onion but is much larger and more subtle in flavour. It is usually trimmed of most of the green tops then chopped or sliced and cooked as an ingredient in stews, casseroles and soups.

mesclun also known as mixed greens or spring salad mix. A commercial blend of assorted young lettuce and other green leaves, including baby spinach leaves, mizuna and curly endive.

mizuna Japanese in origin; the frizzy green salad leaves have a delicate mustard flavour.

mushrooms

button small, cultivated white mushrooms with a mild flavour.

flat large, flat mushrooms with a rich earthy flavour, ideal for filling and barbecuing. Are sometimes misnamed field mushrooms, which are wild mushrooms.

oyster also known as abalone; grey-white mushroom shaped like a fan. Prized for their smooth texture and subtle, oyster-like flavour.

shiitake when fresh are also known as chinese black, forest or golden oak mushrooms; although cultivated, have the earthiness and taste of wild mushrooms. Are large and meaty. When dried, they are known as donko or dried chinese mushrooms; rehydrate before use.

swiss brown also known as cremini or roman mushrooms; are light brown mushrooms having a full-bodied flavour.

mustard

american bright yellow in colour; a sweet mustard containing mustard seeds, sugar, salt, spices and garlic. Serve with hot dogs and hamburgers.

dijon also known as french. A pale brown, creamy, distinctively flavoured, fairly mild mustard.

noodles

bean thread also known as wun sen, bean thread vermicelli, cellophane or glass noodles. White in colour, very delicate and fine; available dried in various-sized bundles. Soak to soften before use.

hokkien also known as stir-fry noodles; fresh wheat noodles resembling thick, yellow-brown spaghetti needing no pre-cooking before use.

oil

olive made from ripened olives. *Extra virgin* and *virgin* are the best, while *extra light* or *light* refers to taste not fat levels.

peanut pressed from ground peanuts; most commonly used oil in Asian cooking because of its high smoke point (capacity to handle high heat without burning).

sesame made from roasted, crushed, white sesame seeds.

vegetable oils sourced from plants rather than animal fats.

onions

green also known as scallion or, incorrectly, shallot; an immature onion picked before the bulb has formed, having a long, bright-green edible stalk.

red also known as spanish, red spanish or bermuda onion; a large, sweet-flavoured, purple-red onion.

pancetta an Italian unsmoked bacon; pork belly cured in salt and spices then rolled into a sausage shape and dried for several weeks before use.

pepitas are the pale green kernels of dried pumpkin seeds; they can be bought plain or salted.

potatoes

baby new also known as chats; not a separate variety but an early harvest with very thin skin.

coliban round, smooth potato with white skin and flesh.

desiree oval, smooth and pink-skinned with waxy yellow flesh.

pontiac large with red skin, deep eyes and white flesh.

russet burbank long and oval, with rough white skin and shallow eyes.

rice

calrose a medium-grain rice that is extremely versatile; can be substituted for short- or long-grain rices.

jasmine a long-grained white rice recognised around the world as having a perfumed aromatic quality; moist in texture, it clings together after cooking.

koshihikari small, round-grain white rice. If unavailable, substitute white short-grain rice and cook using the absorption method.

rocket, baby small peppery green leaf eaten raw in salads or used in cooking.

rolled oats flattened oat grain rolled into flakes and traditionally used for porridge. Instant oats are also available, but use traditional oats for baking.

sauces

barbecue a spicy, tomato-based sauce used to marinate, baste or as an accompaniment to meats.

char siu also known as chinese barbecue sauce; a paste-like ingredient that is dark red-brown in colour with a sharp sweet and spicy flavour. Made with fermented soybeans, honey and various spices.

kecap manis a dark, thick sweet soy sauce used in most South-East Asian cuisines. The sweetness is derived from the addition of either molasses or palm sugar.

oyster Asian in origin, this thick, richly flavoured brown sauce is made from oysters and their brine, cooked with salt and soy sauce, and thickened with starches.

plum a thick, sweet and sour dipping sauce made from plums, vinegar, sugar, chillies and spices.

soy also known as sieu; made from fermented soybeans. Several variations are available; we use Japanese soy sauce unless indicated otherwise.

soy, japanese an all-purpose low-sodium soy sauce made with more wheat content than its Chinese counterparts; fermented in barrels and aged. Possibly the best table soy and the one to choose if you only want one variety.

soy, light fairly thin in consistency and, while paler than the others, the saltiest tasting; used in dishes in which the natural colour of the ingredients is to be maintained. Not to be confused with salt-reduced or low-sodium soy sauces.

sweet chilli comparatively mild, fairly sticky and runny bottled sauce made from red chillies, sugar, garlic and white vinegar.

worcestershire thin, dark-brown spicy sauce developed by the British when in India; used as a seasoning for meat, gravies and cocktails, and as a condiment.

starfruit also known as carambola, five-corner fruit or chinese star fruit; pale green or yellow in colour, it has a clean, crisp texture. Flavour may be either sweet or sour, depending on the variety and when it was picked. There is no need to peel or seed it and they're slow to discolour.

paprika, sweet ground dried sweet red capsicum (bell pepper)

tomatoes

baby vine-ripened truss small vine-ripened tomatoes with vine still attached.

egg also called plum or roma; are smallish, oval-shaped tomatoes.

vinegar

apple cider made from crushed fermented apples.

rice a colourless vinegar made from fermented rice and flavoured with sugar and salt. Also known as seasoned rice vinegar; sherry can be substituted.

wombok also known as peking, napa or chinese cabbage; elongated in shape with pale green, crinkly leaves; is the most common cabbage in South-East Asia. Can be shredded or chopped and eaten raw or braised, steamed or stir-fried.

zucchini also known as courgette.

conversion chart

MEASURES

One Australian metric measuring cup holds approximately 250ml; one Australian metric tablespoon holds 20ml; one Australian metric teaspoon holds 5ml.

The difference between one country's measuring cups and another's is within a two- or three-teaspoon variance, and will not affect your cooking results. North America, New Zealand and the United Kingdom use a 15ml tablespoon.

All cup and spoon measurements are level. The most accurate way of measuring dry ingredients is to weigh them. When measuring liquids, use a clear glass or plastic jug with the metric markings.

We use large eggs with an average weight of 60g.

DRY MEASURES

METRIC	IMPERIAL
15g	½oz
30g	1oz
60g	2oz
90g	3oz
125g	4oz (¼lb)
155g	5oz
185g	6oz
220g	7oz
250g	8oz (½lb)
280g	9oz
315g	10oz
345g	11oz
375g	12oz (¾lb)
410g	13oz
440g	14oz
470g	15oz
500g	16oz (1lb)
750g	24oz (1½lb)
1kg	32oz (2lb)

LIQUID MEASURES

METRIC	IMPERIAL
30ml	1 fluid oz
60ml	2 fluid oz
100ml	3 fluid oz
125ml	4 fluid oz
150ml	5 fluid oz (¼ pint/1 gill)
190ml	6 fluid oz
250ml	8 fluid oz
300ml	10 fluid oz (½ pint)
500ml	16 fluid oz
600ml	20 fluid oz (1 pint)
1000ml (1 litre)	1¾ pints

LENGTH MEASURES

METRIC	IMPERIAL
3mm	⅛in
6mm	¼in
1cm	½in
2cm	¾in
2.5cm	1in
5cm	2in
6cm	2½in
8cm	3in
10cm	4in
13cm	5in
15cm	6in
18cm	7in
20cm	8in
23cm	9in
25cm	10in
28cm	11in
30cm	12in (1ft)

OVEN TEMPERATURES

These oven temperatures are only a guide for conventional ovens. For fan-forced ovens, check the manufacturer's manual.

	°C (CELSIUS)	°F (FAHRENHEIT)	GAS MARK
Very slow	120	250	½
Slow	150	275-300	1-2
Moderately slow	160	325	3
Moderate	180	350-375	4-5
Moderately hot	200	400	6
Hot	220	425-450	7-8
Very hot	240	475	9

index

ARE YOU MISSING SOME OF THE WORLD'S FAVOURITE COOKBOOKS?

The Australian Women's Weekly Cookbooks are available from bookshops, cookshops, supermarkets and other stores all over the world. You can also buy direct from the publisher, using the order form below.

TITLE	RRP	QTY	TITLE	RRP	QTY
100 Fast Fillets	£6.99		Japanese Cooking Class	£6.99	
Barbecue Meals In Minutes	£6.99		Just For One	£6.99	
Beginners Cooking Class	£6.99		Kids' Birthday Cakes	£6.99	
Beginners Simple Meals	£6.99		Kids Cooking	£6.99	
Beginners Thai	£6.99		Kids' Cooking Step-by-Step	£6.99	
Best Food Desserts	£6.99		Low-carb, Low-fat	£6.99	
Best Food Fast	£6.99		Low-fat Feasts	£6.99	
Best Food Mains	£6.99		Low-fat Food for Life	£6.99	
Cafe Classics	£6.99		Low-fat Meals in Minutes	£6.99	
Cakes, Bakes & Desserts	£6.99		Main Course Salads	£6.99	
Cakes Biscuits & Slices	£6.99		Mexican	£6.99	
Cakes Cooking Class	£6.99		Middle Eastern Cooking Class	£6.99	
Caribbean Cooking	£6.99		Midweek Meals in Minutes	£6.99	
Casseroles	£6.99		Moroccan & the Foods of North Africa	£6.99	
Casseroles & Slow-Cooked Classics	£6.99		Muffins, Scones & Breads	£6.99	
Cheap Eats	£6.99		New Casseroles	£6.99	
Cheesecakes: baked and chilled	£6.99		New Classics	£6.99	
Chicken	£6.99		New Curries	£6.99	
Chicken Meals in Minutes	£6.99		New Finger Food	£6.99	
Chinese & the Foods of Thailand, Vietnam, Malaysia & Japan	£6.99		New French Food	£6.99	
Chinese Cooking Class	£6.99		New Salads	£6.99	
Christmas Cooking	£6.99		Party Food and Drink	£6.99	
Chocolate	£6.99		Pasta Meals in Minutes	£6.99	
Cocktails	£6.99		Potatoes	£6.99	
Cookies & Biscuits	£6.99		Salads: Simple, Fast & Fresh	£6.99	
Cooking for Friends	£6.99		Saucery	£6.99	
Cupcakes & Fairycakes	£6.99		Sauces Salsas & Dressings	£6.99	
Detox	£6.99		Sensational Stir-Fries	£6.99	
Dinner Lamb	£6.99		Slim	£6.99	
Dinner Seafood	£6.99		Soup	£6.99	
Easy Curry	£6.99		Stir-fry	£6.99	
Easy Spanish-Style	£6.99		Superfoods for Exam Success	£6.99	
Essential Soup	£6.99		Sweet Old-Fashioned Favourites	£6.99	
Food for Fit and Healthy Kids	£6.99		Tapas Mezze Antipasto & other bites	£6.99	
Foods of the Mediterranean	£6.99		Thai Cooking Class	£6.99	
Foods That Fight Back	£6.99		Traditional Italian	£6.99	
Fresh Food Fast	£6.99		Vegetarian Meals in Minutes	£6.99	
Fresh Food for Babies & Toddlers	£6.99		Vegie Food	£6.99	
Good Food for Babies & Toddlers	£6.99		Wicked Sweet Indulgences	£6.99	
Greek Cooking Class	£6.99		Wok, Meals in Minutes	£6.99	
Grills	£6.99				
Healthy Heart Cookbook	£6.99				
Indian Cooking Class	£6.99		TOTAL COST:	£	

Mr/Mrs/Ms _____

Address _____

_____ Postcode _____

Day time phone _____email* (optional) _____

I enclose my cheque/money order for £ _____

or please charge £ _____

to my: ☐ Access ☐ Mastercard ☐ Visa ☐ Diners Club

Card number | | | | | | | | | | | | | | | | | |

Expiry date _____ 3 digit security code *(found on reverse of card)* _____

Cardholder's name_____ Signature _____

To order: Mail or fax – photocopy or complete the order form above, and send your credit card details or cheque payable to: Australian Consolidated Press (UK), ACP Books, 10 Scirocco Close, Moulton Park Office Village, Northampton NN3 6AP.
phone (+44) (0)1604 642200
fax (+44) (0)1604 642300
email books@acpuk.com
or order online at www.acpuk.com
Non-UK residents: We accept the credit cards listed on the coupon, or cheques, drafts or International Money Orders payable in sterling and drawn on a UK bank. Credit card charges are at the exchange rate current at the time of payment.
Postage and packing UK: Add £1.00 per order plus £1.75 per book.
Postage and packing overseas: Add £2.00 per order plus £3.50 per book.
All pricing current at time of going to press and subject to change/availability.
Offer ends 31.12.2007

* By including your email address, you consent to receipt of any email regarding this magazine, and other emails which inform you of ACP's other publications, products, services and events, and to promote third party goods and services you may be interested in.

TEST KITCHEN

Food director Pamela Clark
Food editor Karen Hammial
Assistant food editor Sarah Schwikkard
Test Kitchen manager Cathie Lonnie
Senior home economist Elizabeth Macri
Home economists Belinda Farlow, Miranda Farr, Nicole Jennings, Elizabeth Macri,
Angela Muscat, Rebecca Squadrito, Kellie-Marie Thomas
Nutritional information Belinda Farlow

ACP BOOKS

Editorial director Susan Tomnay
Creative director Hieu Chi Nguyen
Designer Hannah Blackmore
Senior editor Wendy Bryant
Dietitian Karen Inge

Director of sales Brian Cearnes
Marketing manager Bridget Cody
Business analyst Ashley Davies
Production manager Cedric Taylor

Chief executive officer Ian Law
Group publisher Pat Ingram
General manager Christine Whiston
Editorial director (WW) Deborah Thomas

RIGHTS ENQUIRIES

Laura Bamford Director ACP Books lbamford@acpuk.com

Produced by ACP Books, Sydney.
Printed by Dai Nippon, c/o Samhwa Printing Co., Ltd,
237-10 Kuro-Dong, Kuro-Ku, Seoul, Korea.
Published by ACP Magazines Ltd, 54 Park St, Sydney;
GPO Box 4088, Sydney, NSW 2001.
phone (02) 9282 8618 fax (02) 9267 9438.
acpbooks@acpmagazines.com.au www.acpbooks.com.au

To order books, phone 136 116 (within Australia).
Send recipe enquiries to: recipeenquiries@acpmagazines.com.au

Australia Distributed by Network Services,
phone +61 2 9282 8777 fax +61 2 9264 3278
networkweb@networkservicescompany.com.au
United Kingdom Distributed by Australian Consolidated Press (UK),
phone (01604) 642 200 fax (01604) 642 300 books@acpuk.com
New Zealand Distributed by Netlink Distribution Company,
phone (9) 366 9966 ask@ndc.co.nz
South Africa Distributed by PSD Promotions,
phone (27 11) 392 6065/7 fax (27 11) 392 6079/80 orders@psdprom.co.za

Clark, Pamela.
The Australian Women's Weekly
Food for fit and healthy kids.
Includes index.
ISBN 978 1 86396 579 8 (pbk.).
1. Cookery – Juvenile literature.
2. Cookery (Natural foods – Juvenile literature).
I. Title. II Title: Australian Women's Weekly
641.5637
© ACP Magazines Ltd 2007
ABN 18 053 273 546